faithfully fit

A 40-Day Devotional Plan
to End the Yo-Yo Lifestyle
of Chronic Dieting

CLAIRE CLONINGER
& LAURA BARR

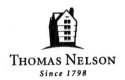

THOMAS NELSON
Since 1798

NASHVILLE   DALLAS   MEXICO CITY   RIO DE JANEIRO   BEIJING

Published by Thomas Nelson, Inc., P.O. Box 141000, Nashville, TN, 37214

All Scripture quotations, unless otherwise indicated, are taken from the New Century Version®. Copyright © 1987, 1988, 1991 by Word Publishing, a Division of Thomas Nelson, Inc. Used by permission. All rights reserved.

Other Scripture references are from the following sources: The Holy Bible, New International Version® (NIV). Copyright © 1973, 1978, 1984 by the International Bible Society. Used by permission of Zondervan Bible Publishers. All rights reserved. The New King James Version (NKJV). Copyright © 1979, 1980, 1982, Thomas Nelson, Inc., Publishers. The Living Bible (TLB), copyright © 1971. Used by permission of Tyndale House Publishers, Inc., Wheaton, IL 60189. All rights reserved. J. B. Phillips: The New Testament In Modern English (PHILLIPS), Revised Edition. Copyright © J. B. Phillips 1958, 1960, 1972. Used by permission of Macmillan Publishing Co., Inc. The King James Version of the Bible (KJV). THE REVISED STANDARD VERSION of the Bible (RSV). Copyright © 1946, 1952, 1971, 1973 by the Division of Christian Education of the National Council of the Churches of Christ in the USA. Used by permission. New American Standard Bible (NASB) © The Lockman Foundation 1960, 1977, 1988, 1995. The Amplified New Testament (AMPLIFIED), copyright © 1958, 1987 by the Lockman Foundation. All rights reserved.

The lyrics to the following songs are reprinted with permission:
"White Flag" (p. 2), by Claire Cloninger and David Baroni, © Word, Inc., 1986. "Spirit Eyes" (p. 32), by Claire Cloninger, © Word, Inc., 1984. "Spirit Wings" (p. 58) by Claire Cloninger and Michael Foster © Word Inc., 1984. "Quiet Hearts" (p. 62), by Claire Cloninger and Kathy Frizzelle, © Word, Inc., 1990. "Time Will Tell" (p. 92), by Claire Cloninger and Billy Smiley, © Word, Inc./Sparrow, 1986. "I Will Choose Your Way" (p. 122), by Claire Cloninger, © Word, Inc., 1990. "You in Me" (p. 152), by Claire Cloninger, © Word, Inc., 1990. "Overcomers" (p. 183), by Claire Cloninger and Morris Chapman, © Word, Inc., 1987.

Library of Congress Cataloging-in-Publication Data:

Cloninger, Claire.
    Faithfully fit : a 40-day plan to end the yo-yo lifestyle of chronic dieting / by Claire Cloninger and Laura Barr.
      p. cm.
  ISBN 10: 0-8499-0988-0 (2006 edition)
  ISBN 13: 978-0-8499-0988-7 (2006 edition)
  ISBN 0-8499-3237-8 (1991 edition)
    1. Dieters—Prayer-books, devotions, etc.—English. I. Barr, Laura, 1952– . II. Title.
  BV4596.D53C56 1991
  242—dc20

Printed in the United States of America

08 09 10 QW 5 4 3

To
John and Spike,
who have loved us whatever shape we were in

contents

acknowledgments

We would like to express thanks, love, and appreciation to the following:

- Our children—Curt, Andy, Ramsay, MacReadie, and David—who have supported us. And when they couldn't support us, at least they tolerated us.

- The precious brothers and sisters who have broken open the mystery of the Word for us during these "formative" years: John Barr, Conlee Bodishbaugh, Paul Sheldon (especially for his teaching on powerlessness), Pam Hanes, Jim Cymbala, and Brennan Manning.

- Our publishers at W Publishing Group, Laura Kendall and Joey Paul, and our very creative editor, Anne Christian Buchanan.

- Our friends and family members who have prayed!

- And especially, Jesus Christ.

a word from claire

This is *not* a book about going on a diet and whipping your poor, pitiful body back into shape. I am weary of diets, and I have deep respect for your body, whatever shape it's in. God made it. That's all I need to know.

Anybody can start a diet. I've started millions of them. Some people even reach their goals on diets. I've done that a few times too. (Well, at least once that I can think of.)

But the people I marvel at are the people who have actually given up dieting: the people who are totally at ease with food; the people who live serene and guilt-free lives from meal to meal, never obsessing about pizza or chocolate chip cookies or calories of any kind. I honestly believe that God created all of us to live like that.

So what happened?

Unfortunately, it seems that humankind's guilt-free association with food was rather short-lived. In the garden, the serpent pointed to the fruit of a certain tree and said, "Aw, go ahead. What's it gonna hurt?" And there we went—all of us!

I guess what I am saying in a roundabout way is that I believe this issue of eating and overeating with which our culture is so obsessed is actually a *spiritual* issue. Some schools of thought would have us believe that it is strictly *physical* and can be handled by decreasing caloric intake and upping the metabolism. That may take care of the problem of pounds, but it doesn't touch the ongoing tug-of-war we have with temptation and guilt. Diets will never solve our problem with food, any more than telling people to "just say no" ever solved our country's problem with drugs.

Newer methods of weight control suggest that we explore *psychological* reasons for our overeating, using everything from self-assessment to group therapy to psychoanalysis. Though discovering "Why?" can be extremely helpful, we are still left with "What now?" and that perennial favorite, "How?"

Behavioral techniques suggest methods for controlling our eating by modifying habits and lifestyle. But even these (which in my experience come closest to effecting change) rely on the strength and motivation of the individual. Personally, I have found that anytime the buck stops with me and everything hinges on my inner resolve and fortitude, I am in big trouble! The harder I try to heal myself, the worse things seem to get!

"So you see how it is: my new life tells me to do right, but the old nature that is still inside me loves to sin. Oh, what a terrible predicament I'm in! Who will free me from my slavery to this deadly lower nature?" These words in the apostle Paul's letter to the Romans (7:23–24 TLB) convince me that what I'm dealing with is indeed a *spiritual* problem. In fact, this verse is a perfect paraphrase for what goes around in my head the day after I've blown another diet.

My own problem with compulsive eating began in high school. It was that insane kind of eating that has little to do with hunger and everything to do with feeling insecure.

Since I also dieted compulsively and was blessed with a

naturally high metabolism, I never developed much of a weight problem. In fact, friends who considered me trim just laughed whenever I tried to confess my shame over this crazy overeating-dieting seesaw I was on. Because I was not fat, they tuned me out and made fun of me for thinking I had some kind of problem. They could not see the feelings of failure, frustration, and guilt I lived with daily.

By now all of us in this country are familiar enough with the various kinds of eating disorders to recognize that weight is not the only indicator of irrational eating. Many degrees and combinations of the anorexia/bulimia nightmare plague Americans.

Many die of these diseases. It is no laughing matter.

For years I, like many others, had been treating my spiritual disorder with physical, psychological, and behavioral remedies. Some brought temporary periods of relief, but none really addressed the core issue.

Perhaps this explains why I believe that what the world needs now is not another diet book full of menus and calorie charts. There are lots of good ones out there—you probably already own two or three. Or another exercise program. There are lots of those too. Or even another scientific solution based on psychological analysis or behavior modification. They line the bookstore shelves.

What we do need, I believe, is a book with *spiritual* foundations—one that will help us stay on the diet—or, better yet, will show us how to eat sensibly and well without needing to call our eating program a "diet." We need a book that will deal with the spiritual issues of diet and exercise—issues that our culture has labeled "motivation" and "willpower"; "incentive" and "perseverance." We need a book that will change our understanding of the spiritual challenges so many of us face in learning to eat well and exercise regularly, that will thereby change our behavior.

We designed *Faithfully Fit* to be this kind of book. You can use it as a companion to any diet or nutrition program or simply as a spiritual motivator toward responsible eating. The daily readings offer hope, courage, challenge, insight, and humor to anyone who is finally ready to stop overeating and start overcoming.

Most importantly, *Faithfully Fit* is not afraid to give spiritual answers to what are essentially spiritual dilemmas. My prayer is that as you read you will be drawn more and more into the knowledge and love of Jesus Christ, the Bread of Life who satisfies our deepest hunger.

—CDC

a word from laura

So, if this isn't a book about the latest diet discovery (and it really isn't), just what is it about? It's a book about healing and wholeness and restoration—*healing* our self-images and our attitudes toward food, becoming *whole* people in Jesus Christ, and being *restored* to his design as children made in his image.

I began this journey toward wholeness by looking in the mirror (not a bad place to start for any of us veterans in the weight/food battle). As I viewed the twenty-plus postbaby pounds I was desperate to shed, I considered the quick-fix options: Crash diet? Liquid diet? Total fast? (These were certainly roads I had traveled before. How depressing! Here I was again.)

And that was when something inside me rose up and refused to opt for the quick fix. That day I realized that the easy way is not really the easy way. It's the hard way, because it has to be traveled over and over again.

I didn't have any professional guidance or input at the beginning. I didn't have any kind of special knowledge or expertise. I started with nothing but a genuine desire to begin eating wisely and exercising regularly. I knew instinctively that what I needed was something long-term and grounded—something that would work from the inside out (from the spiritual me to the physical me). I had tried it the other way around, and I was tired of the old boomerang effect.

I thank God for his perfect timing, for just as I was beginning this journey, my friend Claire was charting a similar course of her own. Together we have pooled our ideas, experiences, and spiritual insights to design a Scripture-based program of action and encouragement for everyone who has had it with the yo-yo lifestyle of the diet-addicted.

Probably none of us would argue with the fact that this is a fallen universe. The Lord's table is spread out before us as a blessing, but Satan is doing his best to turn that blessing into a war zone for many of us. Still, we who have eyes of faith can see our God at work in large and small ways to bring his whole creation back into perfect balance. We are praying that he will use *Faithfully Fit* as a small tool for this purpose in many lives—especially yours!

—LRB

an overcomer's alphabet

A   Ability
(We are able because God is able! Heb. 2:18, 7:25)

B   Being yourself

C   Choosing

D   Doing what you Decide ("Be doers of the word, and not hearers only," James 1:22 NKJV)

E   Eating and Exercise

F   Faith and Forgiveness

G   Grace

H   Hanging on to Hope

I   Integrity

J   Joy on the Journey (not impatient for results, but enjoying getting there)

K   Keeping on Keeping on

L   Listening (to God's still, small voice; to your own decisions)

M   Music

N   New life

O   Others (realizing need for a group and/or a prayer partner)

P   Prayer, Patience, Planning, Point of view

Q   Quiet time

R   Reading and Reflection

S   Serenity, Simplicity, Solitude

T   Thinking and Thanking

U   Unlearning old attitudes and patterns and replacing them with new ones

V   Victory in Christ (already yours, learning to appropriate the power)

W   Willingness to change

X   eXcellence (Christ's call to be your best self)

Y   You (the most important tool—learning to love and accept yourself)

Z   Zest (allowing the Spirit to infuse you with enthusiasm)

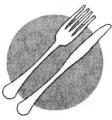

how to use this book

why?

You probably bought this book because you're fed up with diets that don't work, "shape-ups" that don't last, eating and exercise programs you just can't stick to. *Faithfully Fit* is deliberately different. It supplies spiritual motivation and incentives to help you stick with your diet or exercise regimen. Or, if you are not on a diet or specific exercise program, it provides a boost as you strive to eat and exercise in more healthy and responsible ways.

what?

Faithfully Fit offers a six-week program of daily readings, each concluding with a prayer, a Scripture, a Food for Thought section, and optional assignments. You may choose to do all of the assignments or only a few, or you may substitute activities of your own. In fact, we encourage you to do all you can to make this program truly your own. We do suggest, however, that you commit to doing *something* besides just reading through the selection every day. We have found that action—even the act of writing—helps reinforce the positive changes that are happening in our lives.

when?

Use whatever time of day is best for you to do your reading, the assignments, your physical workout, and so on. Your schedule and body clock are not like ours. We may exercise in the morning and do our readings at night. You may do exactly the opposite. With God's help and guidance, you will find the time you need to follow a course that is uniquely your own.

with whom?

Faithfully Fit works equally well for solos, duos, or groups. You may enjoy working through the program with a best friend or a buddy (we did!). Having a prayer and exercise partner as well as someone to confide in can be a real benefit in providing motivation and feedback. We suggest you choose someone who believes in you—someone honest and supportive.

how?

Faithfully Fit is easy to read and follow without any special instructions. But the following pages contain some ideas to help you get started.

how to get started

We suggest you begin preparing for your forty-two-day program at least a week in advance. Being ready to start—physically, mentally, and spiritually prepared—can do a lot to help you finish successfully!

Gather What You Need

You will need a few things, other than this book, to begin the program:

Essential:

❏ *A Bible.* Any translation will do, but we suggest one of the good modern versions, such as the New Century Version.

❏ *A notebook and supplies.* You will also need a loose-leaf notebook with divider tabs, plenty of paper, and, of course, a pencil or pen. We suggest a notebook that is large enough to provide plenty of room for writing, but small enough to be toteable.

Optional:

❏ *Specific diet or exercise program.* Since this program is designed to help *motivate* you to healthy eating and regular exercise, it contains few specifics about *what* to eat or *how* to exercise. You may want to select a sound eating and/or exercise program to use along with this book. A wide array of excellent books, CDs, and videos is available, including many sound Christian programs. But beware of miracle cures and quick fixes; they are the last thing you need to help you get off the dieting yo-yo.

Pick Your Starting Date

We suggest picking a Saturday or other "off day" as your starting date. Mark it on your calendar, and add it to your prayer list.

If you plan to work through *Faithfully Fit* with a partner, get together at least once ahead of time to synchronize your calendars and agree on how you will use the program.

Commit to the Time Frame

As we were planning a six-week program for overcoming overeating, it occurred to us that six weeks works out to almost exactly forty days and forty nights (forty-two, to be precise)! We were immediately struck by the biblical precedent for working within a forty-day framework. Like Jesus, Moses, and other spiritual trailblazers, you will be entering a "wilderness time" of testing, training, and spiritual growth. Carefully consider and prayerfully commit to this "set-apart" period. It can be a special season for you—a time for the Lord to increase as you decrease (in more ways than one)!

Pray

Take time to confess past failures, receive God's forgiveness, and forgive yourself. It's important to start with a clean slate. Make peace with yourself. You need to be in your own corner, not working for the opposition!

Also spend time in prayer asking the Lord to bless your efforts and that what you do will be pleasing to him and beneficial to you. "Remember the LORD in all you do, and he will give you success" (Prov. 3:6).

Prepare Your Notebook

In your notebook, make divider pages for the following six categories:

- *Scripture.* We suggest copying the Scripture passage from the reading into this section of your notebook every day. We have found that writing out the verses helps us enter them into our spiritual "computer." (You may wish to memorize at least one of these verses per week.)

- *Goals.* Goals help us chart our course and evaluate our progress. Your goals may not be totally formed at the beginning, but don't worry. You will be working them out in the first few weeks of the program.

- *Food for Thought.* We have benefited tremendously from copying each day's Food for Thought statement into this section of our notebooks. Reading them over during the week reinforces them. As we accept them into our belief systems, they begin to change our behavior.

- *Journal.* You will be using the Journal section of your notebook to write letters to the Lord—letters that will give you a chance to share your true feelings, insights, requests, thanks, experiences, and so on. Plan to write in your journal at least three times a week. Doing this will keep you honest and open!

- *Insights.* The Insights section of the notebook provides room for you to expound on the *Aha!* moments of revelation that are certain to come from the Lord as you walk with him on this journey.

- *Planning.* In the Planning section of your notebook, you can work out the particulars of your program—the specific ways you will go about reaching your goals. You can work out and record menu plans, exercise schedules, and numbers of miles or repetitions in this section. Some of the assignments in days to come will help you with your planning.

Take an Inventory

Spend some time before your starting date *thinking* in general terms about where you are and what you are hoping to accomplish, both physically and spiritually. You may want to use the questions in the Appendix as a guide.

Record your thoughts in the Journal section of your notebook. Write as much or as little as you care to. But dare to be very honest. The truth will set you free! You may wish to share your inventory with your buddy or your group. Or, if you choose, you may determine that the contents of this notebook will be for your eyes only.

Write Down Some Pre-Goals

A pre-goal is a written statement that helps us get in touch with what we really want for ourselves. Pre-goals begin with phrases such as "I would enjoy . . ." or "I would feel good about . . ." They never begin with "straitjacket" phrases such as "I should . . ." or "I have to . . ."

Pre-goals often evolve into specific goals. For example, a pre-goal such as "I feel much more healthy and alert when I exercise regularly" might become the following specific goal: "I will ride my stationary bike thirty minutes per day."

On the first page in the Goals section of your notebook, write down some pre-goals that come to mind. Try to treat this process like a brainstorming session. There are no right or wrong answers. You're not making any definite commitments yet. Just let your mind wander over some of the benefits of healthy eating and exercise and express your feelings about them.

Get Ready the Night Before

Avoid the temptation to indulge in a "last fling" with food the night before you begin. Instead, eat a light meal and get a good night's sleep. You'll wake up rested and ready to go.

week one: surrender

sur•ren•der (sə ren´ dər), v. 1. to give up possession of. 2. to abandon or relinquish control. 3. to give oneself up, esp. as a prisoner.

Chances are you've tried more than once to be in total control of your eating. And chances are, if you're like most dieters, more than once you've ended up totally out of control.

A good way to begin being *Faithfully Fit* is to surrender the control of your eating to God. He is able to do "much, much more than anything we can ask or imagine" (Eph. 3:20). When we begin really trusting him, he is able to accomplish in us what we have been unable to accomplish in ourselves.

Surrender is not a onetime thing; it is an ongoing process. The Lord is constantly showing us new areas we are holding back from his control. Perhaps eating is for you (as it is for us) one of the more difficult areas to release. Confess this to God, and he will help you begin to let go. We both find a need to surrender our eating to God every morning. In fact, lots of days we have to consciously surrender at each meal!

We suggest that you use Week One as an opportunity to focus on the spiritual discipline of surrender. Find out what it really means to you. How willing have you been in the past to let God be in control? How seriously have you taken your need to allow him to work in you? (Perhaps you've never really tried it before.)

Begin now by looking for ways to make each day more God-directed, especially in the areas of eating and exercise.

White Flag

Chorus:

Lord, I'm putting up the white flag, throwing down my pride,
Wholly and completely sold out to your side.
I'm putting up the white flag; it's what I want to do.
I'm surrendering my whole life,
Surrendering my whole life, Lord, to you.

There's been a battle here inside me ever since I can recall,
Since I heard you asking me to let you have it all.
Now I wonder why I fought you, tried to do things my own way,
When the joy is in surrendering and coming home to stay.

Repeat chorus

Well, it took some time to see it, to really understand
I'm only giving back to you the works of your own hand.
You designed me and you made me to use in your own way,
So I'm trusting you to take my life and use it every day.

Repeat chorus

—Claire Cloninger and David Baroni

day 1: surrender
the problem eater

Who is the problem eater? Is he the fat little fourth grader gobbling Twinkies? Is she the overweight homemaker with an addiction to cheesecake? What about the executive with the soaring cholesterol count, or the bulimic or anorexic teenager who is killing herself to be thin?

The answer is yes. All of the above.

But problem eating extends well beyond these neat stereotypes. There are Americans of all shapes, sizes, sexes, ages, and walks of life struggling with what they choose to chew.

For the purposes of this book, we will define the problem eater as (1) anyone whose eating behavior puts his or her health at risk, (2) anyone whose diet and eating behavior is consistently out of line with what he or she believes is best, (3) anyone who consistently goes against his or her own intentions in the area of diet and nutrition, and/or (4) anyone who is controlled by an obsession with food and dieting.

At times it seems that much of our culture has developed a problem with food. We have been amazed at how many different people—men, women, and teenagers—upon finding out about this book, have commented, "Send me your first copy! I need it!"

3

How can there be one answer for so many different kinds of problem eaters? There are many different approaches to diet and exercise, many schools of thought on how behavior can be changed. But in the spiritual realm the answers are amazingly similar and remarkably simple. And admitting our need for God and surrendering our lives to him and his perfect will for us is always the starting place—the first step to healing any destructive habit in our lives.

Earlier this week we watched a TV special entitled "Deadly Addictions." This program took a comprehensive look at many kinds of addictions, including classic eating disorders, and it included interviews with many recovering addicts. Amazingly, whether the problem was with gambling, eating, sex, or alcohol, almost every addict admitted that the turning point in conquering his or her addiction came as a result of surrendering to "a higher power."

How blessed we are to know our "Higher Power" on a first-name basis! His name is Jesus Christ. He is the one who stands with arms outstretched to each of us, saying, "Come unto me" (see today's Scripture reading).

Whether you have a hundred pounds to lose or ten, whether you have a serious eating disorder or just an old-fashioned tendency toward second helpings—whatever your eating problem, great or small—healing begins when you surrender to the lordship and loving guidance of Jesus Christ. He will lead each of us personally and individually into the way of healing that is tailor-made for us.

—CDC

Prayer

Father, I thank you that you are a God of healing, a God who desires our wholeness and health. Jesus, I thank you for your open arms and your standing invitation to "give all [our] worries" to you (1 Pet. 5:7). I am so weary of this problem with food. And I admit to you that it is something I have not been able to solve on my own. So I surrender, Lord. I cast this problem on you, and I invite you to take over in my life. Fill me with your radiant good health. Help me to want your will for me. I pray in the name of Jesus, Amen.

Scripture

Come to me, all of you who are tired and have heavy loads, and I will give you rest. (Matthew 11:30)

Food for Thought

Jesus is the source of my health and my healing.

ASSIGNMENTS

1. In the Journal section of your notebook, record your feelings about this journey you are beginning. Don't be surprised if you are experiencing a real mixture of feelings: hope, fear, excitement, faith, doubt. When you have finished, imagine yourself wrapping up whatever feelings you have expressed, placing them on God's altar, and surrendering them to him.

2. Chances are, you see yourself as a problem eater. Thoughtfully explore the basic problem you have with food, and enter a simple description of that problem into the Insights section of your notebook.

3. If you have decided to use the buddy system as you go through the next six weeks, try to get together today; if you can't, set a time to do it. During your time together, express hopes, fears, and expectations. Talk about goals and plans. Be sure to begin and end your visit with prayer!

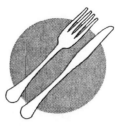

day 2: surrender
the problem is me

When you live on the Gulf Coast, you tend to mark the years of your life by the hurricanes you've endured. I have vivid memories of Hurricane Frederick, one of the most ferocious natural disasters ever to hit Mobile, Alabama. Just in our yard alone, eight trees were ripped out of the ground or snapped off like toothpicks, and two of them came through the roof of our house! Multiply that by the length and breadth and population of a city of 350,000 people, and you're talking about some damage.

There's nothing like a natural disaster to get us in touch with the fact that we're really not as in control of things as we'd like to think we are. I've never felt quite so small and helpless as I did on that September night with the 180-mile-an-hour winds whistling around our house.

But I can name another natural disaster that threatened to do more damage to me, and over a longer period of time, than Frederick ever did. That uncontrollable storm was that of my own selfishness, fueled by the winds of my own ego. As a young wife and mother, I yearned to have a blissful home life and a perfect marriage. And I tried—I really did. But time and again, the storms of my own selfishness threatened to blow my house down!

Looking back on those stormy times, I'm glad that I was forced to face my own powerlessness over myself. For it was this very revelation that let me know my need for God.

English writer G. K. Chesterton must have had something of the same insight in his life. Once, when asked by the *London Times* to contribute an essay on the topic "What Is the Problem in the Universe?" he mailed in this succinct reply: "I am. Sincerely, G. K. Chesterton."[1]

Or as the cartoon character Pogo once wryly observed, "We have met the enemy, and he is us!"

Many of us have spent valuable time and energy trying to deny that the problem is us. We delude ourselves into thinking that if we had a different job, mate, parents, or children, or if we could only move to a different neighborhood or a different town, things would change for the better. That if we had a different figure, body type, or metabolic rate, we would at last be happy.

Real growth begins when we are willing to see that all these circumstances are only externals. Real healing begins when we can at last see ourselves as the problem and the love of God as the answer. Until we come to this crisis of faith, we are dealing only with symptoms. We are putting Band-Aids on cancer. We are rearranging the deck chairs on the *Titanic*.

God cares deeply about our struggle with eating and exercise, but not because he is interested in what size blue jeans we can fit into. He sees our reckless eating as the symptom of a deeper despair, and he wants to heal us. But it is only when we stop denying and start surrendering that he can begin. Only then will we see that outer layer of delusion (and fat) begin to dissolve at last.

—CDC

Prayer

Lord, I know you are showing me where the problem lies. It lies in me. Thank you for helping me come to a place of surrender. I know that I need strength and power beyond myself if I really want to change. Please help me, Lord. I am bundling up all my defenses and rationalizations and excuses and laying them on your altar of love. In faith, I am stepping over that line now and asking you, Lord, to be in control. I surrender to you, Father. In Jesus' name, Amen.

Scripture

What a miserable man I am! Who will save me from this body that brings me death? I thank God for saving me through Jesus our Lord! (Romans 7:24–25)

Food for Thought

Real change can begin when we are willing to see ourselves as the problem and the love of God as the answer.

ASSIGNMENTS

1. During your quiet time, tell the Lord you are willing to stop blaming other things in your life and take responsibility for changing your eating behavior. Thank him for his help.

2. In the Journal section of your notebook, write how you may have been the problem in your own life. Write down any *Aha!* discoveries in the Insights section of your notebook. You may wish to use your journal as a tool for confession.

We can be confident that when "we confess our sins, he will forgive our sins, because we can trust God to do what is right. He will cleanse us from all the wrongs we have done" (1 John 1:9).

3. As you exercise today, be aware that God is with you. Offer your time of exercise as a physical expression of thanksgiving and surrender.

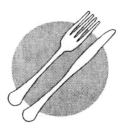

day 3: surrender
a matter of control

I remember when our oldest son, Curt, was a toddler just learning the meaning of "no." One afternoon, while playing outside, he discovered a line of ants busily crossing the front walk. At last! Here was something smaller than he was. He grabbed a stick and, with all the authority of a controlling adult, began shaking it at the ants, shouting, "No-no, no-no, no-no!"

I believe the definitive temptation of our humanity is to try to control our lives—and, at times, everyone else's! Our urge to control began as long ago and far away as the Garden of Eden.

God told Adam and Eve, "Leave it to me. I'll handle the details. You just enjoy. Just name the animals and walk in the cool of the day and that type of thing."

But the serpent told this first man and woman that God was trying to put one over on them—and that they didn't have to put up with it. If they'd just take a tiny nibble of what was forbidden, they could be in control; they could be the gods of their own lives. That sounded good to Adam and Eve. So they bit.

The story of Mary in the Bible is quite different. The angel said to Mary, "God wants to bless you." Mary was a little confused about how that was going to take place. The angel said, "Not to worry. The Holy Spirit will take care of the whole thing, if you're willing." So Mary said, "Let this happen to me as you say!" (Luke 1:38).

Now each one of us faces the same choice. Will we let God do what he wants to do in us, or will we insist on trying to do it—our way? Adam and Eve ended up naked and afraid. Mary ended up filled with God. But choosing Mary's way means being willing to agree with the fact that we're pretty powerless. It means going with God.

The life of Jesus is a model of powerlessness. He chose to divest himself of all power to come to us as a defenseless baby. And at the end of his earthly life, he chose the cross—the ultimate picture of powerlessness. He was nailed up naked, alone, at the mercy of the Romans and the crowd—to the human eye, utterly hopeless. Although the humanity in him struggled against such submission to God's will, in the end, submission was the way he took. He chose powerlessness so that God's power could be shown through him.

So many times, I realize that my struggle with overeating is really a control issue. Where eating is concerned, I want to say, "Nobody's gonna tell me what to do!" But healing can start only when I let go of the reins and stop battling for ultimate authority in my life.

Nobody really loves feeling out of control, but I have learned that agreeing with my powerlessness brings freedom from compulsive behavior. Why? Because it lines me up with the truth of who I am: a created being designed to walk in perfect harmony with my Creator. *Perfect harmony* means he calls the shots and I get a good night's sleep. He leads the way, and I learn how to follow. That's the truth, and it really does bring freedom.

There is also tremendous joy in giving over control of our lives to a loving God. Choosing to die to our own way—our whims, urges, and compulsions—brings us to life in a way we never knew was possible. Admitting powerlessness gets our egos out of the way so God's power can operate in us.

—CDC

Prayer

Father, thank you for your design. Thank you that I don't have to carry the weight of the world on my shoulders. Thank you that you desire to call the shots in my life. And I ask you to take over. I yield the controls of my life to you, especially in my eating. Admitting my weakness, I look to you for strength. You know what is best. Change me from within by the power of your Holy Spirit. In Jesus' name, Amen.

Scripture

Humble yourselves before the Lord, and he will lift you up. (James 4:10 NIV)

Food for Thought

There is tremendous joy in trusting my life to a loving God.

ASSIGNMENTS

1. In the Journal section of your notebook, list all of the areas of your life in which you are willing to admit your own powerlessness. You may wish to include incidents in your past that you can't change, things in your future you do not yet

know, your heritage, your genetic makeup (including height, coloring, IQ, and so forth), any aspect of your looks that you dislike, other people in your life, and your baffling behavior in the area of eating.

2. By now you should be ready to state several specific goals related to eating and exercise—goals to be accomplished during this six-week period. You may wish to discuss them with your prayer partner or group. Write them out in the Goals section of your notebook, and be sure to word them very positively.

3. Consider: compulsive overeating is often a form of rebellion. We like to think that the rules do not apply to us, that we can operate outside the facts and realities of calories, metabolism, and weight gain. When we rebel against controlled eating in any form, we are actually rebelling against rules and authorities, against other people, against ourselves, and against God. What part does rebellion play in your eating problem? Write down your insights in your notebook.

day 4: surrender
inside out

One of my favorite classes in college was Techniques in Musical Theatre. My classmates and I spent a whole semester producing the Cole Porter classic, *Kiss Me Kate*, from casting to curtain call.

We even built the sets, including the elaborate Padua street scene where Petrucio meets and proposes to Katherine. Beginning with nothing more than canvas, boards, and buckets of paint, we ended up with an amazingly authentic-looking slice of old Italy.

We took tremendous care to make each brick and tile and bush look as realistic as possible. Of course, behind the rustic-looking door of Casa Katerina, there was nothing but an empty stage. We had constructed an elaborate façade.

I confess that often I am guilty of doing the same thing with my body. I spend tremendous time and energy on my exterior and far too little time on the furnishings within it. I anguish over dress size and hairdo and makeup and wardrobe, perhaps to cover up the fact that the someone behind the façade is feeling pretty empty.

The world we live in pays great attention to façades. All you have to do is peruse the monthly magazines at any grocery store checkout counter to prove this to yourself. Not only the ads, but the articles, too, instruct the reader in ways to impress others with outer hype.

Scripture informs us that the Lord looks at things from a different perspective. He is much more interested in the interior life than in that brave and made-up face we present to the outside world. "God does not see the same way people see. People look at the outside of a person, but the LORD looks at the heart" (1 Sam. 16:7).

The Lord is not interested in the kind of instant makeovers we find in women's magazines, which refurbish only the façade. Remember the harsh words Jesus used to describe the Pharisees who got all the externals right but neglected the important matters of the heart? He called them "whitewashed tombs" (Matt. 23:27 NIV). He is far more interested in doing an "inside job" on us. He wants to change us at the deepest level of our lives, the feelings and emotions and motives that we frequently hide from each other and even try to hide from ourselves and him.

And here is the beauty of the Lord's interior makeover: when we surrender to him, when we open our doors for him to come in and remodel who we are, we become totally new creations—"Look! I am making everything new!" (Rev. 21:5). The emotional distortions in our lives that caused us to overeat in the first place begin to heal. The old compulsions begin to be tamed. And the tranquil beauty he gives us within begins to affect and transform our outer selves as well.

—CDC

Prayer

Father, thank you for caring more about who I really am than who I pretend to be. Thank you that my façade never fools you, for you know your own creation from the inside out—and you love me anyway! Lord, I give you permission to do an interior makeover on my life. I place myself, my whole personality—motives, emotions, hidden needs, and inner drives—in your hands. Do with me as you will, Lord. I want to be exactly who you designed me to be. In Jesus' name, Amen.

Scripture

But the LORD said to Samuel, "Don't look at how handsome Eliab is or how tall he is, because I have not chosen him. God does not see the same way people see. People look at the outside of a person, but the LORD looks at the heart." (1 Samuel 16:7)

Food for Thought

The Lord is not interested in an instant makeover. When we surrender to him, he comes in and remodels us, inside and out, into totally new creations!

ASSIGNMENTS

1. Have you been overconcerned with externals? Explain how in the Journal section of your notebook. In what areas of your inner life do you discern God at work? Write down any insights that occur to you.

2. As you take your walk (or do your other exercise) today, concentrate on breathing deeply. Ask Jesus to come into your body with each breath you inhale. As you exhale, imagine you are breathing out any qualities or habits you feel he would like to remove from your life.

3. Consider: surrendering to God, both inside and out, is a matter of giving up. Picture a cowboy who has thrown down his pistol and put his hands in the air. The gig is up. Ironically, we who are willing to take this stance and give up to God are the ones who win in the end. Are you still clinging to your old defenses, or are you finally ready to "stick 'em up"?

day 5: surrender
using our resources

When Curt was a baby, we lived for a year in New Orleans on a quaint little street called Bordeaux. The backyard of our very modest duplex just happened to adjoin the grounds of one of the most colossal mansions on St. Charles Avenue. The incredibly lush landscaping of the castlelike stone structure rolled right down to our sparse little plot of St. Augustine grass.

Sometimes during that difficult year when we were struggling to make ends meet, my husband, Spike, suggested laughingly, "Why don't you run next door and borrow a cup of money?" I never actually did it, but it was tempting.

Most of us can look back on lean financial times in our lives. Maybe you're even living through one of them right now. In the midst of the struggle, it's tempting to look across the fence to someone else's greener grass.

But spiritually we need never be in that position. Once we have entrusted our lives to the lordship of Jesus Christ, we fall heir to all of his Father's inner riches. There are no "haves" and "have-nots" in the kingdom. As someone once said, "The ground is level at the foot of the cross." There, all of us are on an equal footing and have equal rights to God's incredible storehouse of spiritual resources.

Why then do I live at times as if I am spiritually bankrupt? Why do I continue to struggle with my compulsive eating when every weapon in God's spiritual arsenal is waiting to come to my defense? Why do I flounder and fret and accept defeat when every ounce of God's power is charged and ready to kick into action at my command?

What kind of power am I talking about? Paul described it when he told the Ephesians: "And you will know that God's power is very great for us who believe. That power is the same as the great strength God used to raise Christ from the dead and put him at his right side in the heavenly world. God has put Christ over all rulers, authorities, powers, and kings" (Eph. 1:19–21).

That is the power available to us in Jesus Christ—exactly the same power that raised Christ from the dead! Surely, then, it must be sufficient power to overcome the relatively minor obstacles in our lives. Surely it is much more than enough power to confront and overcome our daily struggles with overeating. So why isn't it working?

Unfortunately, every time we try to manage the struggle in our own power alone, we forfeit the benefit of his power. When we draw upon only our own meager inner resources to fight our battles, we forfeit the benefit of his resources—the limitless supply of strength, courage, hope, and inner resolve available to us in Jesus Christ.

The spiritual tug-of-war in my life and yours can be won only when we surrender to him and begin to appropriate (lay hold of; seize; own) our inheritance of Spirit power to overcome.

—CDC

Prayer

Lord my God, apart from you, I am a spiritual pauper. I have inadequate energy and resources for fighting my battles, and I often feel defeated. But in you I am rich. I have all strength and hope and power. I am "mighty . . . for pulling down strongholds" (2 Cor. 10:4 NKJV). I surrender to you, Lord. I accept your invitation to become your own child, your spiritual heir. Through faith in Jesus Christ, I now lay hold of my inheritance. I am through trusting in my own willpower. I surrender to you, giving you permission to operate fully in my life. Overcome in me as I am trusting and resting in you. In Jesus' name I pray, Amen.

Scripture

And you will know that God's power is very great for us who believe. That power is the same as the great strength God used to raise Christ from the dead and put him at his right side in the heavenly world. (Ephesians 1:19–20)

Food for Thought

When we start calling on the Holy Spirit power that's available to us in Jesus Christ, we'll start winning our daily struggles with overeating.

ASSIGNMENTS

1. If you haven't already mapped out a plan for regular exercise, begin to do so today, writing out a schedule in the Planning section of your notebook. Be realistic. It is better to begin slowly but be regular about it. Choose something

that is fun and challenging and that will fit into your schedule. If you need help choosing a program, ask at your local Y or health club, or check out one of the excellent videos available on the subject. Personally I love to walk. If you can find a walking partner who has a compatible schedule and is dedicated, that is a great solution. Go for it!

2. Look up and read one of the Gospel accounts of the Resurrection. Express in writing your thanks to God for his resurrection power in your life.

3. Consider: the average American gains one pound per year for every year after the twenty-fifth birthday. Maintaining what we know to be our ideal weight takes work, prayer, and motivation. But it's never too late to reverse the trend!

day 6: surrender
frank's God box

I remember a conversation I had with my sister, Ann, when she was a newcomer to the Christian faith. I had been fretting and worrying about one of my children, trying to nag him into straightening out his life, and this was Ann's helpful comment on my approach: "Claire, I don't claim to know a lot about God, but I do know this much: I'm not him!" That's a pretty good place to begin when it comes to trust.

Once we get out of the business of trying to be all-powerful in our own lives and everyone else's, we give God the freedom to do what only he can do—be God! Tremendous freedom and healing flow into our lives when God is given his rightful place.

Why is there such therapeutic value in giving God our worries? Because tension, stress, and anxiety feed our compulsions. If we happen to be overeaters, they trigger our overeating. But compulsive behavior decreases in direct proportion to the growth of our faith. The worries we trust God to handle cannot act as fuel to our compulsions. An attitude of relaxed faith encourages sane eating habits.

Last week my younger son, Andy, and I discovered a new

way to practice trusting. We were visiting our friend Frank, who is also a new pilgrim on this journey of faith. He showed us a contraption he had rigged up to help him let go of anxiety. He called it a God Box.

By taping the open ends of two Styrofoam cups together, Frank had formed a container of sorts. On the outside he had written with a marker: "Your will, not mine." On one end he had cut a slot.

"Whenever I start worrying or obsessing about anything at all," Frank explained, "I simply write the problem out on a piece of paper and put it in my God Box." His face wore the expression of a child with a new toy! "I just turn the problem over to God and ask him to work out his perfect will in the situation. I've never been this relaxed in my life. It's incredible."

Sometimes it really does help to do something visible, something physical, that symbolizes what we are doing in the spiritual realm. Frank's God Box helped him by giving him a physical way to express the release of his tensions and worries to God.

What problems, stresses, or relationships are causing undue worry in your life right now? Are these things affecting the way you eat? Would it help you to really hand these things over to God?

—CDC

Prayer

Father, I confess my worry as a sin, because it is evidence of my unbelief. I am so tired of being controlled by my fears and anxieties. I long to trust you completely in every part of my life. Help me, Lord, to let go of my stress, my worry, and my desire to control others. Increase my faith, Father. Help me to put my problems and my loved ones into your hands. Help me to let you do what only you can do: be God. Give me that quiet assurance, that inner peace, that releases me from every urge to act compulsively, especially in the area of eating. Keep me in the serene confidence that you are in control. In Jesus' name I pray, Amen.

Scripture

Do not worry about anything, but pray and ask God for everything you need, always giving thanks. And God's peace, which is so great we cannot understand it, will keep your hearts and minds in Christ Jesus. (Philippians 4:6–7)

Food for Thought

Compulsive eating decreases in direct proportion to the growth of our faith.

ASSIGNMENTS

1. Create a God Box of your own design. Use a shoebox, an oatmeal box, or anything you have around the house. The type of box is not important—remember, Frank's Styrofoam cups worked just great!

2. Keep the box on hand during your quiet time. Whenever a person, situation, or thing causes you worry, jot it down on a slip of paper, fold it up, and slip it in your God Box. Confess to the Lord that you have tried unsuccessfully to control or solve these worries. Tell him that you desire his will in each circumstance of life. Do not take it out and

reread it. Every time you are tempted to worry about these things, remind yourself that they are in God's hands. Then praise God again for his faithfulness. When the box is full, burn or throw away your worries, then start over. Note: You may need to write persistent worries or temptations each day and commit them to God on a one-day-at-a-time basis!

day 7: surrender
the right thing

When Bible characters heard from God personally, their experience was sometimes quite dramatic. Moses heard a voice in a burning bush. Paul was struck blind on the road to Damascus. Mary came face-to-face with an angel.

But at other times, such messages from God occurred in everyday ways. Elijah waited on a mountainside, anticipating a thundering voice, and found instead that God's personal word for him was as soft as the whisper of a breeze.

Years ago when our son Andy reached a major crossroads in his eighteen-year-old life, he asked God for a personal word of guidance. God answered him very matter-of-factly, "Andy, you know the right thing to do. Now do it." Andy admitted that the minute he heard those simple and direct inner words, he knew exactly what they meant in his situation.

"I had been knowing 'the right thing' to do for a long time," he confessed. "I just hadn't been doing it."

I believe this is true for most of us most of the time. In almost every area of our lives, God puts within us an unspoken nudge toward doing what we know is right. Unfortunately, though, an unspoken rebellion inside of us nudges us in a different direction.

This is what Paul was talking about in Romans 7: "My own behaviour baffles me. For I find myself doing what I really loathe but not doing what I really want to do. . . . I often find that I have the will to do good, but not the power. That is, I don't accomplish the good I set out to do, and the evil I don't really want to do I find I am always doing" (vv. 15, 18–19 PHILLIPS).

In the areas of eating and exercise, most of us know all too well what is right and healthy. We've read countless books and articles on the subject. We mean to act in our own best interest. Yet, in spite of excellent intentions, many of us find ourselves stuck in behavior that runs counter to what we know is best. Like Paul, we are baffled by our consistently unhealthy choices, and yet changing our behavior seems difficult or impossible.

The slim distance between (a) what we know is right and (b) what we choose to do is the space in our lives that lets us know beyond a doubt that we need a Savior. When our willpower repeatedly fails to deliver us to the right thing in our lives, we cry out like Paul, "Who will save me from this body that brings me death?" (Rom. 7:24 PHILLIPS).

It is at this point that we find the same answer Paul found: "I thank God for saving me through Jesus Christ our Lord!" (Rom. 7:25). Jesus came to earth for precisely this point of despair. His power and love are waiting to bridge the gap in each of us between what we know and what we do. When we come humbly admitting our need and acknowledging him as the source of supply, he empowers us with supernatural strength to do the right thing.

—CDC

Prayer

Father, I thank you for the beautiful paradox of faith. At our weakest and most exasperated, we are closest to the source of true strength that flows from you. Holy Spirit, I pray that you will give me eyes to see my wretchedness and courage to abandon myself into the care and keeping of Jesus Christ. Jesus, I praise you for your saving work on my behalf. I confess to you my sin and rebellion, and I throw myself on your mercy, asking you to save me. I choose your new life over my old one. Infuse me with your power to do what I know is right. I pray in your precious name, Amen.

Scripture

[Jesus] said to me, "My grace is enough for you. When you are weak, my power is made perfect in you." So I am very happy to brag about my weaknesses. Then Christ's power can live in me. For this reason I am happy when I have weaknesses . . . Because when I am weak, then I am truly strong. (2 Corinthians 12:9–10)

Food for Thought

If we let him, Jesus will bridge the gap in us between what we know is right and what we actually do.

ASSIGNMENTS

1. Read Romans 6–8. In your Journal, paraphrase 7:15–25, putting in the specifics of your own life as it relates to your decision to lose weight.

2. There are many points of surrender in our lives once we choose to do what is right in God's sight, including:

- our obsession with food, weight, and appearance.
- our need to be perfect.
- our negativity and our fears.
- our battered self-esteem.
- both successes and failures for God to use or redeem.
- this moment and every future moment.
- our next meal and every future meal, one at a time.
- our own plans in favor of God's plan.

Which of these points of surrender are applicable to your life? What others can you name? In the Insights section of your notebook, write down your personal surrender list.

week two:
point of view

point of view (point əv vyoo ´), n. 1. a specified manner of consideration or appraisal. 2. a mental position or attitude.

Thousands of years ago, the writer of Proverbs wisely said, "Where there is no vision, the people perish" (29:18 KJV). The kind of vision he was talking about, the kind that shapes and changes us from within, grows out of faith. It involves seeing things not as they are, but as they will be, seeing things from God's perspective.

But seeing life as God does isn't easy for us, and God the Father understood our need for visual aids. Jesus became for us a visual portrayal of the amazing possibilities of a life lived in complete union with God. We need no longer wonder what a perfect life would look like. We have seen him!

How does this relate to the matter at hand—the problem of changing our eating attitudes and behaviors? Being transformed from overeaters to overcomers will require a shift in point of view. We must allow God to remove our old images of self-defeating behavior and replace them with *possibility pictures*. We must allow him to give us a fresh outlook, a new hope, an inner image of the new life upon which we now embark.

The second week of meditations, therefore, concentrates on seeing ourselves and our struggle with food from God's point of view.

Spirit Eyes

Let me see you in the battle and not just in the victory,
Let me see you in the darkness and not just in the dawn,
Let me see you in the trial and not just in the triumph,
Let it be your face of love I look upon.

Chorus:
Give me spirit eyes
To see the truth behind the lies,
To find the hope that hides within despair.
Give me spirit eyes
To look behind the world's disguise
And faith to know that I will find you there.

Let me see you in the present and not just in the future,
Let me see you in the sinner and not just in the saint,
Let me see you in the questions and not just in the answers,
Help me find you in the loss and in the gain.

Repeat chorus

—Claire Cloninger

day 1: point of view
changing our focus

It was a bleak January morning. Outside, the sky was still shadowy and gray. I sat alone staring out of the window at our Chinese elm, which stretched its gnarled and leafless silhouette across our deck like the body of an ancient and arthritic giant, twisted and menacing in the half-light, its branches like bare, bony fingers clutching blindly at the misty sky. I could almost hear in my imagination some eerie musical theme in the background.

Then, before my eyes, the scene began to change. Slowly, gradually, the sky behind the elm began to grow golden with the dawn. As it did, my focus shifted. Instead of seeing the dark and gnarled pattern of the tree, I found myself marveling at the intricate design of light that glowed between its branches. It was as though the tree were hung with loops of golden lace that shimmered and glowed in radiant relief against a black backdrop. As the scene changed from darkness to light, the musical theme in my mind began to lift and soar to a triumphant theme.

A teacher in grade school used to say, "It's all in the way you look at things." There's a lot of truth in what she said. As I focused on the twisted branches that January morning, I saw a scene of darkness and dread. Then, as my focus shifted to the light behind the branches, the dreariness I was feeling shifted to hope and joy. Same scene. Two different perspectives.

Very often, life is like that. We are not affected so much by what is actually happening in our lives as we are by how we choose to interpret what is happening. We can look at our circumstances through eyes of despair and negativity, or we can shift our spiritual focus to one of hope, joy, and gratitude.

More specifically, we can view our daily struggle with overeating as a tedious, difficult, boring inconvenience that robs us of pleasure. Or we can make the conscious choice to view it as a physical and spiritual challenge through which God is giving us an opportunity to grow in our knowledge and trust of him.

If we let him, God will use every one of our difficult circumstances to mold us into his perfect design. Once we have grasped that reality, we can thank God for our struggles . . . and surrender them to him. That's when we'll begin to see the patterns of light behind whatever the darkness in our lives may be.

—CDC

Prayer

Father God, forgive me for focusing so often on the dark side of my circumstances. I choose today to focus on all that is hopeful and positive about where I am right now. Give me a clear spiritual perspective that sees the light of your love behind the darkness. Help me to see my struggle with overeating as a way to know you better and trust you more. Thank you for using my weaknesses to make me strong in you. Amen.

Scripture

You are all people who belong to the light and to the day. We do not belong to the night or to darkness. (1 Thessalonians 5:5)

Food for Thought

I choose to view the days of this spiritual eating and exercise program as an opportunity to grow in my knowledge and trust of God.

ASSIGNMENTS

1. Think of a situation you are facing. Practice focusing on the positive side of it by writing, in the Journal section of your notebook, two separate descriptions of this situation. In the first description, paint the situation as bleakly as possible. Rewrite the same scene, purposely emphasizing whatever is optimistic, lovely, and/or hopeful about it.

2. Write a list of all of the positive aspects about adopting moderate and healthy eating and exercise habits as they relate to you. State them in the present tense. For example: (1) "I feel so much better physically when I am eating healthy food in moderate amounts." (2) "I feel more confident when I know I'm at a healthy weight for my body." Record your list in the Insights section of your notebook.

3. Begin your mornings this week by stretching thoroughly. Lie in bed a minute or two before getting up and stretch each part of your body: legs, arms, neck, shoulders, even

ankles and fingers! When your feet hit the floor, you'll feel much more supple and ready to go. Don't forget to stretch before and after your exercise routine, too.

day 2: point of view
a God's-eye view

Several years ago we bought a very used car for our teenage sons—an AMC Spirit that we lovingly dubbed "the Spirit." Permission for excursions was granted that year by saying, "Yes, you may go . . . *if* 'the Spirit' moves you" (which frequently it did not!).

For some reason this morning I was thinking about the maddening day I spent at the courthouse trying to weed through a tangle of red tape in order to get the Spirit registered. It was worth all the frustration, because that was the day I learned an important lesson about getting "a God's-eye view" of things.

I was into my second half-hour, standing in my third line, fuming with impatience at a painfully slow typist behind a huge, gray electric typewriter.

Just as I was considering choking her with her own typewriter ribbon (in Christian love, of course), I heard the Lord's still, small voice. "See the woman behind the typewriter?" he whispered.

"Yes, Lord," I answered.

"I love her."

"*Her?*" I questioned. Surely we weren't looking at the same person!

"Yes, her," he assured. "She is my child. Try seeing her as I do."

Oh well, I thought. *Since I'm going to be here till Jesus comes back anyway, I might as well give it a try.*

I looked her over. With my own eyes I saw a perfectly plain, fairly dumpy gray-haired lady who was inconveniencing me. *Nothing especially lovable here,* I thought.

And then it happened. As I watched her, I prayed, "Let me see her as you do, Lord," and she began to be transformed before my eyes. I saw the plump but graceful fingers making their deliberate way across the typewriter keyboard as she cheerfully did her job in the face of our grumbling. I saw the perfectly symmetrical gray waves of her hair rising and dipping across her head and converging neatly on the nape of her neck. I saw the way her eyebrows arched above her lowered eyelids like tiny teepees. *Wow,* I thought. Then I pictured her looking in the mirror every morning as she dressed to come to this thankless job.

Suddenly I was flooded with an amazing warmth as I felt the tender love of our Father come through me to her. *What a treasure she is!*

The real miracle, of course, is that he loves each one of us with the only-child tenderness that I felt for the gray-haired typist. He sees us as precious and unique and thoroughly lovable. He cherishes and values each of us more than we can ever fully know.

How much better we would be to ourselves if we could catch a God's-eye view of our own lives. We would not hurt our own feelings with negative self-talk or stuff our own bodies with harmful amounts and kinds of food. We would daily be about the business of nurturing ourselves because we would know that we are valuable in the eyes of our Father. We are his treasures!

—CDC

Prayer

Oh, Father, I praise you for the tender love you have for me. Thank you that I am a unique treasure in your sight, Lord. Help me to capture and keep a vision of who I am to you. Help me to allow that vision to transform the way I live. Let me make every decision in light of the way you cherish and value me. Help me to choose healthy foods in moderate amounts to nourish this body of mine, remembering that you designed me in love. In Jesus' name, Amen.

Scripture

Read Psalm 139 to help you get in touch with God's special love for you as an individual. Copy your favorite verse into the Scripture section of your notebook.

Food for Thought

If we could catch a God's-eye-view of our own lives, we would not hurt our bodies by stuffing them with harmful amounts and kinds of food. We would daily be about the business of nurturing ourselves because we would know that we are God's treasures.

ASSIGNMENTS

1. In the Journal section of your notebook, write a love letter to yourself as though it were from God, paraphrasing some of the ideas found in Psalm 139. Write out a list of specific ways your life can change once you get a God's-eye view of yourself. (For example: "I will take better care of my body, knowing it is valuable to God.")

2. During your exercise time today, be aware that God is with you, delighting in your presence. Use this time as a chance to talk things over with him. Thank him again for his love.

3. Consider: someone wise once said that God loves and accepts us exactly as we are and where we are, but he loves us too much to leave us there. We grow strong as we practice looking at ourselves through the lens of his love and acceptance rather than through our own perspective of harshness and criticism. I find I have more success "loving" my extra pounds away than judging them away. Once I have accepted my excess pounds as part of who I am, they are more likely to melt away.

day 3: point of view
the joy of exercise

I suffered through PE in school, always feeling woefully inadequate at anything athletic. I looked for as many easy ways out as possible—always selecting the sport that required the least exertion and the position on the team that required the least skill. I had the idea that exercise was something I had to suffer through and get over with as soon as possible. It never occurred to me that it could bring joy!

Looking back, I see now that one of the main problems was my unfortunate tendency to compare myself to others. Comparison is almost never helpful. In the beautiful old meditation "Desiderata," the writer points out that there will always be someone better than you are and someone not as good. In either case, when you compare, you are stuck with an attitude problem. Either you feel inadequate and inferior or puffed up and proud. Neither spiritual condition is conducive to inner tranquility.

I can remember only one time in my life when indulging in comparisons led me to a positive insight. In fact, I consider my insight on this particular day a milestone in learning to enjoy exercise. Let me share it with you.

I was jogging near the lake in the municipal park near my

house, struggling with the heat and my own lack of energy. My legs felt like five-hundred-pound weights, and my breath was coming in short, labored puffs. Just as I was crossing a small bridge, I saw a stately American egret spread its wings and lift its body up out of the shallow waters where it had been wading. As I watched the egret soar overhead, I felt myself, by comparison, to be a clumsy, plodding, thoroughly inadequate physical specimen. I plodded on, feeling dejected.

Then, rounding a curve, I saw something that gave me a totally different perspective. In front of one of the houses across from the park, a woman was patiently assisting her elderly mother down the walk to the car. The older woman was using a yellow dinette chair for a walker and painfully, laboriously progressing, inches at a time. My heart went out to her. A simple thing like walking had become a painful ordeal.

Suddenly, I felt as light and graceful as the soaring egret by comparison. I could feel my feet almost flying beneath me. I thanked God for my body, just as it was, with all of its capabilities and its limitations.

Each of us has something to be thankful for. If we can move at all, that is a blessing. This week, thank God for the privilege of exercising, and ask him to help you discover its joy!

—CDC

Prayer

Father, I'm so thankful for my body just as it is, with all of its pluses and minuses. Lord, I commit my body now to you, asking you to help me find or design an exercise program that will be perfect for me and my needs. Help me to enjoy the privilege of moving and exercising, never taking it for granted. And finally, Lord, I ask you to help me begin to accept myself and see my body as your workmanship, precious in your sight. In Jesus' name, Amen.

Scripture

And so, dear brothers, I plead with you to give your bodies to God. Let them be a living sacrifice, holy—the kind he can accept. When you think of what he has done for you, is this too much to ask? (Romans 12:1 TLB)

Food for Thought

Each of us has something for which to be thankful. If we can move at all, that is a blessing. Thank God for the privilege of exercise, and ask him to help you enjoy it.

ASSIGNMENTS

1. If you are using the buddy system, share with your friend the exercise plan you formulated last week. Pray for each other every day this week as you continue to carry it out. You may even wish to do your walking, aerobics, or whatever you have chosen to do together.

   If you are doing this program on your own, explain your exercise plan to one other person and ask for prayer support.

2. Consider: we who struggle with overeating are definitely

not alone. Many thousands of us are trying to change our appearances and/or behaviors. An estimated eighty million people are trying to stay on a diet in the United States this very minute![1]

3. As you progress in your exercise program, an excellent boost for your muscles and your spirit is a massage. If you've never had one, you are in for something special. Nothing I can think of makes me feel more relaxed or in tune with myself physically. Many YWCAs have someone trained in giving massage, or your local physical rehabilitation center may be able to recommend someone. Discover one of the joys of exercise—treating yourself to a good rubdown!

day 4: point of view
expect a miracle

Ten years have passed since my first visit to the little church by the ocean, but my memories of it remain fresh and vivid. The first thing I noticed on that summer Sunday long ago was not the building, but the people. They arrived early. They greeted each other warmly and moved to their seats with a real sense of anticipation. The whole church was alive with the feeling that something truly amazing was just about to happen.

And sure enough, it did. This worship service made me feel as if I had come home! The music was beautiful; the prayers were powerful; the love was almost tangible. There were pockets of silence for experiencing God's Word and a sermon that really reached into my heart.

But what impressed me most was the last thing I saw as I left the building that day. There was a sign hanging just above the door. Stark white lettering on a red silk background spelled out just three simple words: "Expect a Miracle." I don't know why it hit me so hard, but I actually walked out of there with heart palpitations!

I thought about that sign for days. And one thing became clear to me as I reflected on its message: the people who worshiped at the little church by the ocean had definitely been practicing what had been preached that Sunday. They had arrived expecting something wonderful, and they had not been disappointed.

In my own Christian journey, I have come to realize that expectation is closely linked to faith. To pray for help or healing or deliverance and then plod on my way without expecting any kind of change is a faithless way of praying. And yet I confess that I have found it easier at times to expect God's healing and deliverance for other people in other areas than to expect it for myself in the area of eating.

Low expectations inevitably seem to draw low results. When I expect to yield to the temptation of a delectable dessert, of course I do. When I expect eventually to fail at any diet I begin, my failure is as good as accomplished. People say we can expect to add a few pounds a year as we grow older. And guess what's been happening?

Well, I'm fed up (pun intended)! I've had it with low expectations and poor results. I'm ready to lift my eyes and expect that miracle! I need God's help and healing and deliverance. And I know he is as ready to deliver me from this kind of bondage as he was to deliver Joseph or Daniel or Paul in the Bible. I know it will take a miracle to keep me faithful to healthy eating and disciplined exercise—and that's exactly what I'm expecting! Are you with me?

—LRB

Prayer

Father, you are the Creator and Author of all good gifts. Thank you that you hold out in your hands an offer of new life and power in the name of your Son, Jesus. I pray now, Jesus, that you will give me new expectations, great expectations! Thank you that it is not by my own strength, but by your power, that this is possible. Come, Holy Spirit, and work a miracle in me. I anticipate it with gratitude, and I give you the glory. Amen.

Scripture

The whole creation is on tiptoe to see the wonderful sight of the sons of God coming into their own. (Romans 8:19 PHILLIPS)

Food for Thought

Expectation is closely linked to faith. The Lord is ready to deliver the help you need. Expect it!

ASSIGNMENTS

1. Review the pre-goals and goals you have been working toward. In what way has your focus shifted? If necessary, reword your goals. Evaluate your progress.

2. Stretch your expectations by picturing your heart's desire in the areas of eating, nutrition, and fitness. How will it feel when God has had his way in your life? How will you be different? (Try to imagine and describe what it will really be like.) Write down your answers to these questions in the

Journal section of your notebook. Date this journal entry and seal it with a prayer in Jesus' name.

3. Consider: expectation is an outgrowth of faith. The Bible describes faith as "knowing that something is real even if we do not see it" (Heb. 11:1). It means believing—and acting—before we see the proof with our eyes. It is an inner sense of knowing something's so. It is a quiet assurance that tells us the thing we are praying for is already coming to be!

day 5: point of view
a portrait of possibility

One of the best Christmas gifts I ever gave my husband was a large acrylic portrait of our two sons and me. Softer and more impressionistic than a photograph, it brings back memories of that year when they were two and four years old in much the same way that a half-remembered dream lingers long after you're awake. It's all there in soft colors and nostalgia: The serious look on Curt's little freckled face. Andy's mouth slightly open and that dreamy expression in his eyes. And there I am seated between them, minus the laugh and frown lines, looking every inch the competent and adoring mom.

My favorite part of the portrait is my hands. When we sat for the artist, she had me fold my hands loosely and comfortably in my lap. Those hands give me such a peaceful look. My portrait seems to be saying, "Motherhood? It's a piece of cake! Noise? Confusion? Fighting? Daily demands? Hey, I can handle it. I'm cool, calm, collected. I've got it under control. I'm the mom here. I can cope!"

On many a hectic day when the boys were growing up, feeling totally rattled by the everyday chaos, I walked through the living room and caught a glimpse of my portrait. There I was on canvas, peacefully poised, confidently smiling, with those softly curved hands at rest.

Hey, that's me, I reminded myself. *I'm the mom in this situation. I can handle it.* Then I felt something inside me calm down and regain composure. How I loved that painting. It was more than art to me; it was a visual tranquilizer!

Who said "A picture is worth a thousand words"? There's a lot of truth to that. Being able to flesh out an idea with a physical image adds tremendous power to the idea. And a mental image, when it is pictured in detail, can be as powerful as one seen with the eyes.

In my ongoing journey toward healthy eating, what mental picture of myself am I rehearsing? Am I picturing in my mind's eye all my past failures at trying to eat well? Or am I allowing the Lord to form a new image within me of a God-controlled person who is able to enjoy the freedom of making wise and healthy choices? Am I able to picture the beautiful and gradual changes that are already coming into my life as I keep my feet steadfastly on the path the Lord is laying out before me?

—CDC

Prayer

Lord Jesus, I thank you for beginning to create within me a beautiful picture of who I can be in you. You are showing me qualities of character that I never before associated with myself. I thank you for each brush stroke you are adding to this inner portrait. Thank you for painting in all of the patience, hope, humor, courage, discipline, trust, and confidence that I will need. Keep this portrait of possibility vividly and colorfully present in my mind's eye as you begin to make the picture a reality in my life. Thank you most of all, Lord, that when I look closely I can see that my portrait is becoming the very image of you! I pray in your name, Amen.

Scripture
We are being changed to be like him. This change in us brings ever greater glory, which comes from the Lord, who is the Spirit. (2 Corinthians 3:18)

Food for Thought
God will help you form in your mind's eye a picture of who you can be in Christ as you change your way of eating and exercising. This will help you leave behind old habits and behavior patterns.

ASSIGNMENTS

1. Today you will be using words to paint a *possibility portrait* of yourself. Ask the Lord to give you a vivid picture of all you will be as you allow him to lead you into more healthy eating and exercise behavior. Picture yourself enjoying the physical benefits of a more attractive appearance. See yourself enjoying exercise, sleeping soundly at night, making new friends, and so on. Describe the picture in detail in your Journal.

2. Try working out to one of the excellent Christian exercise videos or DVDs that are available. Or put your favorite CD in your Walkman and step outside.

3. Another body and soul booster is exercising to Scripture memory CDs.

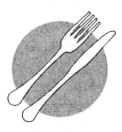

day 6: point of view
food as obsession

My whole life I've heard the proverb that states, "As he thinketh . . . so is he" (Prov. 23:7 KJV). In other words, we are what we think about. If this is true, I have spent much of my life as a pizza.

But seriously, folks, I would not even dare to calculate the number of leisure hours I have logged thinking about food—what I know I should eat today, what I shouldn't eat but am really hungry for, what I have eaten and wish I hadn't, what I resisted eating but wish I'd given in to. *Ad nauseum.*

One of the most obvious but often overlooked facts about the food-obsessed person is that he or she can often become a big-time bore. Life is full of so many wonderful, interesting, thought-provoking things that it is surely a crime to waste so much precious time on this planet thinking about food.

Didn't Jesus himself say, "A person lives not on bread alone" (Matt. 4:4)? And wasn't he also the one who said, "Surely life is more important than food, and the body more important than the clothes you wear" (Matt. 6:25 PHILLIPS)?

Jesus was not suggesting that food is not necessary. (Who knows better than he that food is essential to our lives? After all, he was around when human life was thought up and brought into being, and he is certainly acquainted with all that is required to keep it going.) He was saying, however, that food is not a worthy focus for our hearts. If we just seek God with our hearts, he will take care of the other things (such as food) that he knows we need.

> Don't worry and say, "What will we eat?" or "What will we drink?" or "What will we wear?" The people who don't know God keep trying to get these things, and your Father in heaven knows you need them. Seek first God's kingdom and what God wants. Then all your other needs will be met as well. (Matthew 6:31–33)

I think back to one summer at church camp when I shared a cabin with a girl I'll call Marsha. She was an attractive girl who made good grades and was musically talented. But kids our age ran from Marsha like the plague. Why? She was a nervous wreck of a food fanatic who counted the calories in every lettuce leaf. Her repertoire of conversation topics consisted of dieting and exercise—period. She didn't have time or energy left over for friends or friendships. Her total life focus was on chewing, digesting, and metabolizing food. Consequently, she was a lonely, miserable, and driven girl, worried and old before her time.

Thinking of Marsha's sad little life puts me in mind of something my daddy used to say to us: "Nobody ever had a nervous breakdown worrying about the other fellow." People who are willing to spend a healthy share of their spiritual energy caring about the pain of others will not have room in their hearts for unhealthy self-obsession.

Perhaps it's time to face the fact that food has become an

obsession. If we are willing to change the focus of our hearts, God is more than willing to help us. His words to us clearly mark the road to healing: "Brothers and sisters, think about the things that are good and worthy of praise. Think about the things that are true and honorable and right and pure and beautiful and respected . . . And the God who gives peace will be with you" (Phil. 4:8–9).

—CDC

Prayer

Father, forgive me for the amount of precious time I have wasted obsessing about food, calories, exercise; my weight, my body, and my looks. I need a new perspective, Father. I long to be able to see life from your point of view—valuing what you value and taking the rest in stride. Free me, Lord, to care deeply for others, to recognize and respond to their pain. Release me from this prison of self-centeredness so that I can enjoy the beauty you have put all around me. In Jesus' name, Amen.

Scripture

Think only about the things in heaven, not the things on earth. (Colossians 3:2)

Food for Thought

The person who is obsessed with food, calorie counting, dieting, and so on is destined to become the person who is self-centered, boring, and lonely. If you have become that person, the Lord wants more for you. Allow him to change the focus of your heart and mind.

ASSIGNMENTS

1. Read and paraphrase Philippians 4:5–8. In your Journal section, write your paraphrase in the form of a prayer ("Lord, help me to . . .").

2. Consider: one good way to deal with "food on the brain" is to determine to outlast it. Usually a compulsion to eat is short-lived. Postpone gratifying it for thirty minutes, and you'll almost always find the desire has diminished. An added benefit is that you will be strengthened each time you are able to outlast the compulsive urge.

3. It is helpful to face and replace negative body feelings. Consider one woman's expressed feelings about her body:

When I feel fat, my vision becomes skewed. My perception of reality completely changes: I see only fat or thin. I compare myself to every slender woman in the grocery store, the bank, the gas station. I stare at bodies in my dance class and wonder what they eat and how their thighs can stay so slender. My sense of myself is vague; I'm not sure who I am. Feelings and words and actions lose their crispness, their definition. I move slowly, as in a stupor. I apologize for myself over and over.[2]

If you relate to any of this, ask the Lord to heal your obsession with your weight. Ask him to replace your negative feelings about yourself with his positive view of who you are in him. Ask him to show you the beauty he sees in you, and ask him to give you courage to set healthy weight-loss goals without being obsessive.

day 7: point of view
the need to look up

love it when the Lord uses the things closest at hand to teach me his truth. Case in point: an incredibly beautiful spring morning. I'm sitting outdoors, hunched over little scraps of paper and trying to pull a teaching on praise and worship out of the abyss of my foul mood.

Then from somewhere inside of me a silent voice says, "Look up!" And in the natural beauty right around me I find a million amazing reasons to praise the one who made it all. Fragile new blades of grass. Leaves in every shade of green imaginable. Azaleas in almost-gaudy pinks and purples. Birds and butterflies everywhere. And I had wasted most of a morning looking down!

The Lord who loves us is always calling us to look up. He is always drawing us out of ourselves, to him. He longs to give us his perspective on problems and to elevate our spirits as well as our outlooks.

As we are learning new habits in the areas of eating and exercise, we would do well to heed his freeing call to look up. Rather than becoming bogged down in thoughts of what we "should" do and "ought" to do, we can gaze upward at the one who gives us grace to overcome in ways we never thought possible. Rather than staying stuck twenty-four hours a day in the humdrum particulars of low-cal menu plans and calorie charts, we can be lifted by looking at the one who is over and above all things.

When I think of the spiritual advantage in looking up, I always think of Peter walking on water. As long as Peter kept his gaze firmly fastened on Jesus, he had the power to stay on top of the waves. Looking down caused him to sink. We, like Peter, do well to keep focused on what God is able to do through and for us rather than looking down at our potential failures and defeats.

I love the words to a song that Claire wrote for Joni Eareckson Tada's second album, *Spirit Wings*. When we look up, we are given "Spirit wings" for overcoming.

Now when my life confines me, I just look to you,
And soon my heart is soaring high above.
Troubles look much smaller from your point of view,
Lifted up on Spirit wings of love.

Spirit wings, you lift me over all the earthbound things,
And like a bird my heart is flying free.
I'm soaring on the song your Spirit brings.
O Lord of all, you let me see
A vision of your majesty;
You lift me up, you carry me, on your Spirit wings.

—LRB

Prayer

Father, I pray that you would place your loving hands under my chin to keep my eyes always lifted to you. I thank you, Lord, for your glory and your grace that put in perspective my worries about what I eat and how I look. I choose today to be your child and to receive from you all that I need to be a whole and healthy person. In Jesus' name, Amen.

Scripture

I lift up my eyes to you, to you whose throne is in heaven. (Psalm 123:1 NIV)

Food for Thought

We are so much more than mere bodies. By looking up we focus on the one who made us. We stay in touch with the spiritual dimension of who we are in him and we are strengthened and encouraged to take care of these bodies with which he has gifted us.

ASSIGNMENTS

1. Today, purpose to look up many times—both spiritually and physically.

2. As you refer to your schedule of commitments for the day, deliberately plan to view each from a different perspective. "Look up" at what God is showing you in each situation. Enjoy nature, the people you are with, and the insights you receive as you go through your day. Think less about rushing and achieving and more about living and delighting.

3. As you exercise today, concentrate on finding things to enjoy. The music? The natural surroundings? Your exercise companion? The feeling of satisfaction as you stretch and work your body? Let go of the sense of obligation you feel about exercise and view it as a gift you are giving yourself.

4. Consider: when we view our lives through a lens of self-will, we get a narrow perspective. Our faith in God gives us a broader view; we look up and out. And we learn to see that life is more than just surviving. We discover the fulfill-ment of serving others, and we celebrate the joy of his life in us.

week three: prayer

prayer (prâr), n. 1. a spiritual communion with God. 2. an earnest request.

Many people live with the impression that Christianity is basically a set of rules and regulations by which to live. It's not! Christianity is a relationship. It is the only religion, in fact, that is based on a relationship with a person—the person of Jesus.

Like any relationship, our relationship with the Lord will grow only as we spend time with him—talking and listening; sharing our thoughts and feelings, doubts and desires; waiting for the loving touch we feel when we know he has heard and that he cares.

As we walk through this journey of overcoming overeating, the relationship we have with him is everything. Our prayer time is the time we focus on taking off the old nature and putting on the new. It is the time we meet with God so that he can bring about the changes that are necessary for us to become—among other things—wise and healthy eaters. The transforming friendship that grows during our prayer times will be the key to our becoming all he would have us be.

This week's meditations are designed to help draw you into a deeper life of prayer. They include ways to pray and things for which to pray. Hopefully they will inspire you to seek time in his presence and to receive all that he has for you as you commune with him.

Quiet Hearts

Your silence falls like rain upon our thirsty souls
As we leave our busy lives behind.
Your presence fills our emptiness, and as it does,
We wonder at the simple peace we find.

Chorus:
Quiet hearts, you speak to quiet hearts.
Quiet words you whisper in a still, small voice.
Quiet hearts, you come to quiet hearts,
And in your perfect peace we can rejoice,
For, Lord, you make your home in quiet hearts.

Amazing how your Word can heal us from within
When we come and yield ourselves to you,
We find we're filled with songs of worship once again,
For in the silence love has made us new.

Repeat chorus

Bridge:
And now we can return to life's demands
With energy and passion for the day,
For in the silence you reach out your hand
And lift us up to live a life of praise.

Repeat chorus

—Claire Cloninger and Kathy Frizzelle

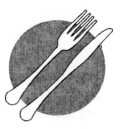

day 1: prayer
praying the way

With all the things I don't know about healthy eating (and there are many, for I am still very much in the learner category), one thing I *do* know: the only way I am going to get from out-of-control to consistently wise eating is down the path of prayer.

If the Word is daily spiritual food, prayer is the enzyme that digests that food and applies it to our lives. Prayer is the exercise that transforms spiritual food into spiritual muscle so we can do daily battle with the challenges and temptations that confront us as we strive to change our habits and behaviors.

Prayer turns a belief into a relationship. Again, Christianity, when it's working, is a relationship—with the one who has the answers and the power we lack. Every functional Christian life is built on prayer.

Here are some concrete ways to get your prayer engines revved up and keep them going:

- Most important, be regular in prayer. Go to God *every* day, sometimes several times a day—definitely before each meal. You will enter his presence, where strength, wisdom, and discernment are free gifts.

- Be specific in your requests and desires. Nothing is too small or insignificant. Remember 1 Peter 5:7: "Give all your worries to him, because he cares about you."

- Ask God to give you a goal weight—the right weight for you—whether you are trying to lose, gain, or merely maintain.

- Ask daily for the desire and the power to eat right. You have to want to want it. God can take a mustard seed's worth of desire and turn it into a life-changing motivation! And remember, his grace comes in daily packages.

- Seek his wisdom. Ask him to show you what to change in your daily circumstances in order to bring about his will for you. Stick to his wisdom instead of your own (Proverbs 3:5: "Don't depend on your own understanding").

- Commit yourself—including your struggles with overeating—to the Father in prayer. Especially commit yourself to a godly understanding of your body and of food.

- When you blow it, confess quickly. "We can trust God to do what is right. He will cleanse us from all the wrongs we have done" (1 John 1:9). Guilt often causes us to overeat, so deal with it immediately!

- Be willing to cry out to God when you are feeling desperate. Crying out was a common prayer stance for men and women in the Bible, from the prophets to the disciples. Be willing to holler "Help!" when you need it. God will show up every time.

—LRB

Prayer

Father, thank you for delighting to hear my voice, and for desiring a relationship with me. As I enter into times of communion with you, clear away all the things that would distract me and keep me from you. I love you, and I want most of all to walk as your child. I pray in the power of the name of Jesus, Amen.

Scripture

Ask, and God will give to you. Search, and you will find. Knock, and the door will open for you. Yes, everyone who asks will receive. Everyone who searches will find. And everyone who knocks will have the door opened. (Matthew 7:7–8)

Food for Thought

When the God of the whole universe is available and more than willing to help you do what is good for your body and your life, surely it is a wise thing to take advantage of his help. Call on him today!

ASSIGNMENTS

1. Look up Romans 8:26 and copy it into your journal. How can the contents of this verse help to shape your prayer life? Be specific.
2. A walk on your own is a wonderful opportunity for prayer (in addition to being good exercise). You may wish to jot down names or key words relating to prayer concerns on a slip of paper. Carry this with you to jog your memory as you go.

3. Before making any food choices this week (whether at the grocery store, a restaurant, or your refrigerator), make a point to stop and pray. Ask the Lord to empower you to make choices that are healthy for you and pleasing to him.

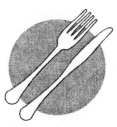

day 2: prayer
the heat of the battle

Some days, by the time I turn out the light and put my head on the pillow, I feel as if I've been in a battle. There's a very good reason for this: I have!

Our daily lives are a battleground of sorts, but the Bible warns us that the war we're fighting is a spiritual one. Paul cautioned the church at Ephesus that "our fight is not against people on earth but against the rulers and authorities and the powers of this world's darkness, against the spiritual powers of evil in the heavenly world" (Eph. 6:12).

If this seems a little too spooky to apply to real life, think about it this way: What are the things that really get us down? What are the enemies that really sink our spiritual ships? Aren't they those subtle ideas and feelings that creep in unbidden and cause us to get off track or give up altogether—feelings like depression, low self-esteem, or discouragement?

Physical weapons won't do a thing for us against enemies of this kind. Did you ever try giving a karate chop to a bout of depression, or a knuckle sandwich to a feeling of despair? It simply doesn't help. To fight spiritual enemies, we need spiritual weapons.

God has supplied us with a whole arsenal of weapons,

beginning with a full suit of armor that protects against every onslaught. There is a belt of truth, a breastplate of righteousness, shoes of good news, a helmet of salvation, and the sword of the Holy Spirit itself, which is the Word of God (see Eph. 6).

The wisest thing I can do during times of temptation, as I'm trying to change my eating habits, is to suit up every morning in this spiritual armor. I marinate my mind in the good news of God's true Word. I remind myself and my unseen enemies of who I am in Christ: I am a child of God, saved by grace, washed by the blood of Christ, and filled with the power of his Holy Spirit. In me is the very righteousness of God in Christ Jesus (Rom. 3:21–22). And I can remind my enemies that when Christ is my dwelling place, "no weapon that is used against [me] will defeat [me]" (Isa. 54:17).

Of course, the ultimate weapon in our spiritual arsenal is prayer. Prayer can turn a demure homemaker, a mild-mannered accountant, or an innocent schoolgirl (anyone, in fact—man, woman, or child) into a powerful warrior. When we pray empowered by God's Spirit, we become "mighty . . . to the pulling down of strong holds" (2 Cor. 10:4 KJV).

I have become convinced in my current struggle to overcome negative eating that thirty minutes of prayer a day will do more for me than twenty-four hours of struggling and fighting in my own strength. We win battles of this kind by praying, trusting, and standing in God's power.

—CDC

Prayer

Father, I thank you for equipping me to do battle against the subtle attacks of the enemy. Give me wisdom and discernment to recognize as enemies those feelings and ideas that pull me off course and hinder me from following you. Give me the courage and determination to stand on your promises and to persevere in prayer. As I daily put on your armor, give me victory in your name. Amen.

Scripture

We do live in the world, but we do not fight in the same way the world fights. We fight with weapons that are different from those the world uses. Our weapons have power from God that can destroy the enemy's strong places. We destroy people's arguments and every proud thing that raises itself against the knowledge of God. We capture every thought and make it give up and obey Christ. (2 Corinthians 10:3–5)

Food for Thought

The ultimate weapon in our spiritual arsenal is prayer. Thirty minutes of prayer in the name of Jesus every day can build powerful spiritual muscle!

ASSIGNMENTS

1. In your Journal, write down each piece of spiritual armor listed in Ephesians 6 and its purpose. Reread your list every morning this week. As you dress each morning, be conscious of putting on the pieces of God's armor.

2. If you're using the buddy system, be sure to use your buddy as a prayer partner. Check in with each other several times a week to make prayer requests and receive prayer reports. Even if you're going through the program on your own, we suggest you find a friend to pray for you as you continue. Prayer is the most effective agent of change we know.

day 3: prayer
power in numbers

In our culture, heroes most often are the strong, silent, solo types—from the Robinson Crusoes of times past to the TV and movie heroes of today. Americans admire, even idolize, those who have learned to go it alone in this big, bad world—who make their way with little or no assistance from anyone.

It makes good fiction, but it's not a lifestyle I'd recommend. Medical researchers, insurance companies, and sociologists have all come to the conclusion that people are healthier when they are not alone. God knew that from the genesis of who we are. He designed us with an innate need for one another.

We who have begun this journey toward healthy eating can gain a special benefit from companionship. There is power in numbers. Having a group to share with and be accountable to can make all the difference in the world as we strive to change our behavior. Having one or more special friends with whom we share prayers, hopes, failures, and encouragement can be invaluable.

What are some times that you might benefit from having a buddy in your corner? A buddy is invaluable in helping to fight what I call the "silent sabotage" that washes over us when we're least expecting it. In case you're wondering, silent sabotage comes in many varieties. Here are a few:

1. You are doing great on your new eating regimen, and you're feeling fantastic about yourself. Suddenly you hear a little voice in your head that says, "You know it'll never last. It's just a matter of time before you're back on the Twinkies. Might as well give it up now. Why postpone the inevitable?"

2. While cooking supper, you realize you've been tasting the spaghetti sauce liberally—probably over a hundred calories' worth! How discouraging! A feeling of hopelessness sweeps over you that says, "Well, today is blown. You might as well eat whatever you want."

3. You have finished the big report you've been working on for two weeks. What a high! You deserve a fantastic reward. You feel an overwhelming urge for rocky road ice cream.

SOS! This is the time for a buddy. Someone who knows you and knows what you've got invested in changing your old patterns. Someone who can pray with you to defeat the silent sabotage of the enemy. Someone who encourages you to hang in there and stands by you while you do.

Scripture shows us time and again that there is spiritual strength in groups, especially when it comes to prayer. Jesus promised, "I tell you that if two of you on earth agree about something and pray for it, it will be done for you by my Father in heaven. This is true because if two or three people come together in my name, I am there with them" (Matt. 18:19–20).

A buddy is a prayer partner and much more. She's someone

you can trust, someone who doesn't put you down. A buddy is fun to exercise with; eat a salad with; shop for a new, smaller size dress with; and celebrate a five-pound weight loss with (by seeing a movie, not eating a banana split!).

Where do buddies come from? Your church, your exercise group, your office, your Bible study group, your neighborhood. If you don't already have one, I'm praying that you'll find a buddy this week! (Of course, one of the best things about having a buddy is *being* a buddy to someone else!)

—CDC

Prayer
Father, I thank you for designing us with a need for one another. Help me to find a group of people with whom I can share and to whom I can be accountable. Help me also to find that special buddy on whom I can depend and with whom I can be real. And, Lord, I do thank you for being that kind of friend to each of us. Thank you for your promises that you will be with us always, that you will never leave us nor forsake us. Thank you that I'm never alone. In Jesus' name, Amen.

Scripture
A friend loves you all the time. (Proverbs 17:17)
There are friends who pretend to be friends, but there is a friend who sticks closer than a brother. (Proverbs 18:24 RSV)

Food for Thought
Scripture shows us time and again that there is spiritual strength in numbers. There is nothing strong about being too

afraid to admit your need. Consider asking the Lord to lead you to someone you can share and pray with, a true buddy.

ASSIGNMENTS

1. If you have decided against the buddy system, write down the names of friends or acquaintances who might be willing to share this journey with you on a less-regular basis. Spend some time considering and praying about how to build support into your eating and exercise program. If you feel you would benefit from a group, look up the names, addresses, and phone numbers of weight-loss programs in the Yellow Pages. Spend some time researching those in order to find the right one. (Note: Some churches have Christ-centered weight-loss programs.)

2. If you do have a buddy, and you haven't shared your goals and pre-goals with each other, take time to do so this week. Ask your buddy to suggest ways for you to stay on course.

3. Sometimes a supportive friend is able to see good things in you that you cannot see. When you meet with your buddy or share your program with a friend, make a point of affirming each other in writing. List specific positive qualities. Keep your buddy's list of your good attributes handy in your notebook to refer to when you need a boost!

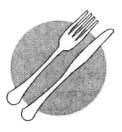

a prayer "skeleton"

Long ago, someone taught me to use the acronym ACTS as a prayer outline of sorts. The letters stand for four components of prayer—Adoration, Confession, Thanksgiving, and Supplication—and they suggest a helpful progression for the prayer experience. For years now these four words have supplied me with a framework—a "skeleton," if you will—upon which the body of my prayer life has been supported.

Though I have used the ACTS method for years, I only recently thought of using it to pray specifically for my eating habits. What a powerful weapon it has become in my struggle to eat sanely! Join me for my quiet time and see what I mean:

Adoration first. Early morning on an ordinary winter Wednesday. The abrasive buzz of the alarm clock pries my eyes open and sets my mind scurrying through the morning agenda: school day . . . breakfast . . . lunchboxes. I groan internally, resenting the fact that my struggle with food has to begin at the very crack of dawn!

Stumbling to my favorite quiet-time chair, I begin to formulate what I have to offer the Lord in prayer. A phrase comes into my mind from a favorite hymn: "For you are my God." Turning these words to him, I realize that God, not thoughts of food, should come first! I begin right then to adore him, to look lovingly at him, to worship (derive my "worth-ship" from) him.

Next, confession. From this vantage point, my sin is easy to see: my disordered priorities, my preoccupation with gift over Giver. I begin by confessing those things specifically, and from that beginning comes the awareness of my powerlessness over these areas of sin. I confess that too.

Now, thanksgiving. Feeling forgiven makes the heart thankful! I begin to get in touch with God's incredible mercy and faithfulness. I thank him. I see his gifts to me: my health, my strong (though slightly rounded) body, the grace of living in a time and place where too much food can even *be* a problem! How blessed I am!

Finally, supplication. (Having adored, confessed, and thanked, the things I ask for are more likely to be in line with God's will than if I had moved immediately into the "gimmes.") I ask him to come first in everything all day, especially in my food decisions. I pray for self-control and strength to resist temptation. I ask him to be at the heart of all I do in relation to food, from choosing to chewing!

My ACTS "skeleton" has put power in my willpower, added gratitude to my attitude, and taken pounds off of my person. It comes to you free of charge and highly recommended!

—LRB

Prayer

Father, thank you that your help comes to us in many forms. Thank you for helping us to pray, and thank you for your Spirit who prays through us. I want to pray according to your will, adoring you for who you are, confessing my sin readily and humbly, thanking you for your many blessings, and asking for your help and direction in all things. Put into my heart the desire, the time, and the way to develop this life of prayer. In Jesus' name I ask it, Amen.

Scripture

Always be joyful. Pray continually, and give thanks whatever happens. That is what God wants for you in Christ Jesus. (1 Thessalonians 5:16–18)

Food for Thought

Adoring God, confessing failures, expressing thanks, and asking that he meet your needs (in that order) is a good progression for a healthy prayer life.

ASSIGNMENTS

1. During your quiet time today, write out the words *Adoration, Confession, Thanksgiving,* and *Supplication.* In the Journal section of your notebook, describe what these four words mean to you. During your prayer time, either write out your prayers under these headings or use them to order the things you pray.

2. In which of these four areas do you feel you are weakest? Which is hardest or most confusing for you? Using a concordance, you may wish to do a word study on this area.

3. Find a picture of yourself when you were at your goal weight or a picture in a magazine that inspires you to action. Put it on your refrigerator as a constant source of motivation.

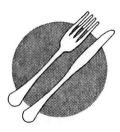

keeping short accounts

Okay, you blew it. With the best of intentions and a couple of good days under your belt, you got off the phone (a not-so-pleasant conversation with your child's teacher) and went directly for the cookies. To top off the guilt you were feeling over being an ineffective parent, you added the guilt of failing yet once again in the eating-correctly department.

By that time it was late afternoon, almost suppertime, so you figured you might as well just "hog it up"—bread with butter, dessert, all the extras that guaranteed to make your transgression a real fall from grace. Later in the evening, you began thinking that you would have to start over tomorrow anyway, so why not treat yourself to one last splurge—a midnight snack! Finally, as you turned out the light, it occurred to you that this was already Thursday, so you might as well wait until Monday and really blow out the whole weekend.

How many times have you and I followed that familiar path to defeat?

Actually, as much as I hate to admit it, what I've described is a true-life documentary of a recent episode of my own. Only this time, thank the Lord, something good came of it. For once, with cookie crumbs still on my lips, I sat down sadly and thought about what had started it all. A feeling of failure, for which I had tried to compensate, had been the culprit. And my unwillingness to confess it had compounded the damage.

Matthew 5:25 says, "Agree with your adversary quickly" (NKJV). In other words, be quick to say to the Lord, "Father, I admit my shortcomings, and I confess my sin."

We are all going to blow it from time to time. It is important to keep short accounts because "if we confess our sins, he will forgive our sins, because we can trust God to do what is right. He will cleanse us from all the wrongs we have done," (1 John 1:9). We don't have to go on filling our feelings of emptiness and inadequacy with food. The Lord will immediately give us a clean slate, and we can begin again—not tomorrow or Monday or after Christmas, but right now.

So how about it? Today, why not open your account books to him? Let him clear the liabilities column. And be willing, at a moment's notice, to do it again!

—LRB

Prayer

Father, I thank you that the death of your Son on Calvary paid the price for me. Forgive me for constantly overlooking this and taking matters into my own hands. It doesn't work. I lay before you now those things that are separating me from you. I ask that you, in your mercy, forgive and restore me to you. Only in you do I find healing and victory. Yours is the power and the glory! Amen.

Scripture

Copy Matthew 5:25 into your notebook and personalize it: "I agree with my adversary." Then copy 1 John 1:9. This one deserves to be memorized!

Food for Thought

Whenever we confess, God is just waiting there to forgive us, and he does!

ASSIGNMENTS

1. Consider the past twenty-four hours and ask God to show you where you have blown it in any area of your life. Write these down and, after asking for God's forgiveness, write the word *Forgiven* over each entry. Tear the page out of your notebook and throw it away.

2. Are you still worrying about any unfinished business from the past? Do you know that if you've asked for forgiveness, God has long since forgotten it? As a wise Bible teacher once told me, "God puts our sins in his lake of love and puts up a 'No Fishing' sign." If any old sins or failures keep surfacing in your own mind, picture yourself tying a rock to each old offense and sinking it in a huge, blue lake. Remind yourself that they are gone for good.

3. Try adding a little extra oomph to your exercise program. If you're walking, you may wish to add fifteen to thirty minutes

to your walk—or try carrying some light weights. If you're in an aerobics class, try adding that extra effort that gives you a stronger workout. But don't overdo it; it's much better to build over a period of time than risk injury with a single all-out effort!

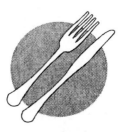

day 6: prayer
seeking solitude

Yesterday I wrote a paragraph in my journal. Rereading it today, I added an enthusiastic "Amen!" in the margin. I think I may be on to something!

Help me not to fear the solitude you call me to each day, but to flee to it. Help me to see that you are moving me into life-enhancing experiences if I will just cooperate with your grace and stop straining against the current of your will for me. You want to save my life—my real life, not this false, self-conscious, compulsive shell. You want to save the me that is really you-in-me. But to get to the real me, you must strip away this shell of fears and fantasies and fickle distractions. The preoccupations with working and eating and seeking the approval of others. Somewhere underneath this gaudy outer garment is the serene beauty of the possible me. How I yearn toward that reality, O Lord. But first I must be still and let you operate.

For centuries Christians have known that surrendering to Christ in times of quiet, prayerful solitude is the way of healing and wholeness. And for as many centuries, Christians have strained against the simple discipline of solitude because everything in the world seems to go contrary to our efforts to be still.

Those of us who struggle with compulsive overeating (as with other unwanted and compulsive behaviors) have much to gain from seeking solitude. Nothing emasculates the power of a compulsion like routinely removing ourselves from people and all the preoccupations that go with them.

The solitude I am describing here, however, is not the same as withdrawing ourselves from others when we feel left out or inferior. That kind of aloneness, sometimes referred to as "isolating," is usually destructive rather than helpful. It can even lead the overeater to a food binge based on self-pity.

Nor am I talking about trying to fight our battles alone without the help and support of others. Exaggerated self-reliance can set us up for failure—especially if going it alone means going without God's help too.

The solitude that heals is not a "running away" but a "running to" someone. It is a purposeful, seeking time—sitting at the feet of the Lord, surrendering our problems to him, listening for his still, small voice. It is a time for letting the uptightness of daily life spin itself out. It is a way to reach and draw from the well of serenity that waits for every seeker after solitude.

Jeanie Miley describes her own daily journey into solitude in the book *Creative Silence*. This prayerful "pilgrimage" yielded many spiritual benefits for the author, including a breakthrough in the area of overeating. Miley speaks of enclosing her day in "parentheses of surrender" as she retreats from her noisy world, morning and night, to hear God's voice.[1]

Henri Nouwen, speaking of personal transformation in his

book *The Way of the Heart*, says that "solitude is the furnace in which this transformation takes place."[2] As we seek the Lord in the solitude of our hearts, we are brought more and more into a place of healing and wholeness.

—CDC

Prayer
Lord Jesus, how blessed I am to be invited to spend time in your presence. Thank you for the healing that is available to me if I will seek you in the silence. Sow in my heart the seed of solitude—a longing to draw away from the crowds and turn toward you. Make a path through my heart's distractions so that I may get through to where you dwell . . . then let me hear from you. Touch me, heal me, mold me into the healthy, whole person you would have me be. In your name I pray, Amen.

Scripture
Do not change yourselves to be like the people of this world, but be changed within by a new way of thinking. Then you will be able to decide what God wants for you; you will know what is good and pleasing to him and what is perfect. (Romans 12:2)

Food for Thought
In Psalm 46:10, the Lord calls each of us to be still and know that he is God. In the stillness we are in a wonderful position to begin to know who he really is.

ASSIGNMENTS

1. In your Journal section, write out the benefits of solitude as they might apply to your own life. Describe times (if any) that solitude has been a major factor in your spiritual growth. List obstacles that stand in the way of finding time alone, and suggest ways for overcoming each. For instance: "Obstacle: telephone interruptions. Possible solution: take phone off hook for thirty minutes during baby's naptime."

2. Buy or check out a Christian book on the subject of prayerful solitude (for example, the two books mentioned in this meditation). Begin reading it, asking God to help you apply its truths to your life.

3. In the Planning section of your notebook, make a list of possible times that you could take twenty to thirty minutes for personal solitude. Select the most promising time and commit to it every day for a week. Enter it into your calendar and honor your commitment to yourself.

gratitude for food

I remember one January 2 when I was bound and determined to start my New Year's diet. I had cleared the refrigerator of all remnants of holiday goodies and had gone to the grocery to stock up on healthy foods. I walked in the front door carrying my groceries and spied on our foyer table a decorative tin box from a local pecan company that someone had left as a gift. I recognized the box immediately, and I knew without looking that it contained one of my major weaknesses—roasted pecans.

I can tell you that my dominant emotion at that moment was not gratitude for the gift. Just having roasted pecans on the premises was a threat to my every good intention.

In spite of the fact that we claim to love food, most of us who overeat have developed an adversarial relationship with food. Because we have found the struggle to control our eating behavior so difficult, we have learned to view food as our enemy. We fear it; we resent it; we cower at its power!

In truth, food is a gift from God that is basic to our survival and essential to our well-being. Food, along with every other created thing, is something God regarded in the creation story told in Genesis 1 as "good" and even "very good." He intended food for our enjoyment and sustenance, yet we have come to regard it as a threat, a source of pain, confusion, disorder, and disobedience. What a lie! Food is not to blame. Food is not our enemy.

We do have an enemy, though. The Bible describes him as a liar, as the one who twists and distorts reality, the one who takes what God intended for our good and uses it as a weapon against us.

We will not be free from overeating until we recognize the lie that Satan has sold us and acknowledge what is true (John 8:32: "Then you will know the truth, and the truth will make you free"). Food is not our enemy, but our ally. And it cannot control us, either. In fact, in the first two chapters of Genesis we see that God put us humans in control of food, not the other way around. A roasted pecan cannot jump out of a tin box and force me to eat it! I have nothing to fear from food.

The Lord can heal my distorted perception of food when I come to him in prayer. I can begin to see food as a gift from God and stop giving it power in my life. With an attitude of gratitude, I can begin to give God praise and thanksgiving for his gifts and receive food as the blessing he meant it to be.

—CDC

Prayer

Father, I praise and thank you for the gift of food. Thank you for your daily provision of food for me and my loved ones. Help me, Father, not to take that gift for granted. Help me to view food as you would have me to—not as an enemy but as an ally, provided for my nourishment. Jesus, I ask you to heal any misconceptions or warped notions I may have acquired about food. Give me the discernment to recognize the lies of the enemy. Give me a grateful heart. I pray in the strong name of Jesus, Amen.

Scripture

Now may the Lord of peace give you peace at all times and in every way. (2 Thessalonians 3:16)

Food for Thought

With an attitude of gratitude, I can begin to give God praise and thanksgiving for his gifts and receive food as the blessing he meant it to be.

ASSIGNMENTS

1. Reread 2 Thessalonians 3:16. Then write it out in your Journal, putting the words in the first person and applying the prayer to yourself personally. Add the following phrase at the end of the prayer: "especially as I eat slowly and appreciatively."

2. Consider: it takes nearly twenty minutes for your stomach to register the fact that you have eaten and feel satisfied. Eating slowly gives your body a chance to catch up with your taste buds and your awareness a chance to catch up with your appetite. Eating slowly and thankfully is not only spiritually sound and socially correct; it is an excellent and easy way of taking in less food and thereby gaining less weight!

3. If weekends are a high-temptation time for you, make a point to plan something special for this weekend that doesn't involve food. Hiking, biking, photography, museums, and movies are excellent choices. A drive in the country can yield

new experiences. Or plan a trip with a friend to a nearby town to check out the shops and activities available there.

4. Beginning today, at every meal, sit quietly for a moment before eating, looking with appreciation at the food you have put on your plate. Don't immediately grab it and attack it like a dreaded foe! Consider the color and texture and contemplate the vitamin content. Then bless God our Provider for each thing on your plate by name. Realize what a gift your food is, and what an ally! Eat slowly and appreciatively.

week four: patience

pa•tience (pā´ sh̯əns), n. 1. the quality of bearing misfortune or pain without complaint. 2. calm tolerance of provocation or delay. 3. perseverance or diligence.

Patience is an undervalued virtue in the present day. We live in a society that demands instant gratification in almost every area of life—including eating. Fast-food restaurants stand on every corner to make certain that no one goes hungry, even for a moment.

Too often in our struggles with overeating we have sought a short-term cure when what we needed was long-term healing. This week we ask you to focus on the virtue of patience. We ask you to look at the big picture, concentrating on lasting changes rather than quick fixes.

Patience is a virtue born out of faith. And faith is a gift. We pray that God will grant you the faith to slow down and start trusting him as God of the long haul—the Alpha and the Omega who was and is and is to be, the "forever principle" in your life!

Time Will Tell

Lord, I can see
I'm not yet what I should be,
And yet your love's changing me.
Slowly I find
You touch my heart and mind;
In time, I know I will see
The life of grace you have placed inside of me.

Chorus:
And time will tell
That love will finish what it starts.
Time will tell
All you've hidden in my heart.
Lord, I know so well,
Only time will tell.

I'm not afraid;
I'm learning how to wait
On love that never comes late.
Time takes its time,
And with your life in mine,
I find, I'm closer each day.
And in a while, I will see you face-to-face.

Repeat chorus

Second chorus:
Time will tell
That love will have the final say.
Time will tell
Where there's faith, you'll find a way.
Lord, I know so well,
Only time will tell.

—Claire Cloninger and Billy Smiley

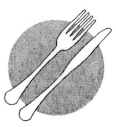

day 1: patience
can't we just fly?

Recently we were driving down a state highway on our way home from a family vacation. The car was packed! Two adults, three children (one under two), and three weeks' worth of clothing, sporting equipment, baby necessities, and assorted other gear. The word *sardines* comes to mind.

As we passed the two-mile mark of what was to be our second four-hundred-mile day, a little voice queried from one of the piles of paraphernalia, "Can't we just fly?"

I suppose I could have answered that question logically. ("Flying is too expensive, and we'll need the car when we get there.") But I decided it was really more of a plea for the quickest and easiest way out of a torturous situation than a real question in need of an answer.

How many times have I, at the beginning of yet another diet or exercise plan, heard that same little voice inside my head: *Can't I just fly?* I want to get from here to there the fastest, easiest way. Never mind the cost (to my body) or what I'll need when I get there (a different heart attitude). I just want to get the trip over with!

This is a book of daily meditations for a very good reason. We are on a journey that must be traveled one day at a time. (Sometimes even one hour or one minute at a time!)

There is no quick way to get from this weight to that, from this size to that, or from this bad habit to a better one. Reading the last chapter first will not give the instant gratification we all want. Skimming the table of contents will not yield three quick and easy shortcuts to help us lick this thing once and for all.

The Lord gives us *this* day our daily bread. Accept it gratefully. Put aside tomorrow and the next day and the next. Stop hurrying. Relax into this moment. Experience it. Breathe deeply, and learn to trust God in the *now*.

We may not be able to soar in the physical sense, but when we learn to patiently do things in God's time, he lifts us up on Spirit wings, and we are airborne after all (see Isa. 40:31)! He gradually changes us "to be like him. This change in us brings ever greater glory" (2 Cor. 3:18).

Remember how precious you are to the one who made you. Stay on the journey with him, one day at a time. And he will be faithful to bring you to your destination in the fullness and grace of his time.

—LRB

Prayer

Father, thank you for being in this with me for the long haul. You never give up, and you never get in a hurry. You are eternal, and you are eternally faithful. Help me today to receive the daily bread you have for me. Help me to experience the joy you have for me when I walk in obedience to your leading. Bring to my mind and heart, Father, over and over, that you are my destination and that, in you, my getting there will be perfect. Thank you, Lord. Amen.

Scripture

But the people who trust the Lord
will become strong again.
They will rise up as an eagle in the sky;
they will run and not need rest;
they will walk and not become tired. (Isaiah 40:31)

Food for Thought

Remember how precious you are to the one who made you. Stay
on the journey with him one day at a time. And he will be faithful to bring you to your destination in the fullness and grace of
his time.

ASSIGNMENTS

1. In your Journal, write a prayer or a personal reflection relating today's Scripture to your own specific needs.

2. If you have been finding it difficult to establish or maintain
   a daily time with the Lord, make your time with him a priority this week. God works in us when we patiently and
   persistently seek his life and his strength. Use your time
   with him for reading the Bible, reading the daily meditations from this book, writing in your notebook, talking to
   the Lord, and listening for his word to you. Perhaps you
   will need to set your alarm clock an hour earlier in the
   mornings. An early time of quiet reflection is a way of gath-
   ering strength for the battles in the day ahead.

3. This week, review the goals you have set and begin breaking them up into smaller goals. We reach almost all worthwhile goals by accomplishing a series of smaller ones. For instance, someone whose goal is to serve on the city council doesn't set that goal one day and get elected the next. The process of reaching that goal takes months, during which time she works toward the smaller goals of filing for the election, putting together an election committee, raising funds, drumming up support, and formulating her position on important issues. In the same way, our eating and exercise goals are ones we reach in small, achievable increments. Working toward and achieving small goals along the way helps us move ahead steadily without becoming discouraged. A weight-loss goal of eighty pounds or an exercise goal of running a marathon are almost too far in the future to keep in sight. Small goals we could set in advance of those overall goals might be:

- I will average two pounds a week until I have reached my ultimate weight-loss goal of eighty pounds.

- I will participate in the five-kilometer fun run at the park on Labor Day.

- I will be able to fit in a size _____ pair of running tights by Christmas.

The joy of achieving these incremental goals will do a lot toward giving you patience for the long haul of meeting your overall goals.

the miracle cure

Suppose there were headlines in tomorrow morning's paper stating that a well-known scientist had finally invented that long-awaited miracle cure for weight control. For a minimal fee of five thousand dollars, this device, an incredible Body-Weight Regulator, could be safely implanted into the human brain.

The amazing regulator, acting as an internal weight thermostat, would trigger brain waves leading its recipient to choose the most nutritious and personally satisfying food for his/her unique needs. The regulator would indicate the ideal time to begin a meal as well as the precise time to stop eating. Statistics as to each person's body type, metabolic rate, and so on, could be programmed into the regulator so that there would never be a moment of doubt or indecision in choosing the proper amount and kind of food for each situation.

How many people do you think would be calling their surgeons the very next day to schedule an implant? Diet books and programs, calorie counters, even scales would all be obsolete. Everyone would have to have a Body-Weight Regulator implant!

Would it surprise you to know that such a system has already been invented? It has. Would it surprise you even more to know that there is one implanted in your brain and mine? There is. God Almighty, the great Creator of humankind, installed just such a system in every single human being. It is standard equipment on every model!

The indication given for the ideal time to eat is known as *hunger*. Actual physical symptoms are triggered within the brain to let each of us know that now is the time. The indication that it is time to stop is the feeling of being comfortably full (not stuffed). Scientific studies have even proved that a body will naturally seek the foods containing nutritional elements it is lacking. (For instance, I remember an example in my high-school science book about a child who kept eating chalk at school. She was found to have a deficiency of calcium, which the chalk contained.)

Unfortunately, many of us in this country have allowed our amazing internal weight regulators to fall into disuse. We were raised in a culture that uses the clock as the signal to eat rather than allowing the hunger meter to do its job. In fact, we use every other eating cue in the book as a signal to chow down. We eat because we are bored or angry or lonely or depressed. We eat because we're happy or relieved or feel like celebrating. Every reason but being hungry.

Many of us, too, keep eating well past the comfortably full signal our bodies are trying to give us. We eat our way into the stuffed-to-the-gills category. And some of us have done this so long we don't even recognize the signals anymore. (If you are in doubt as to whether you are actually hungry, it's pretty safe to assume that you are not! Hunger is a real, deep emptiness accompanied by stomach growls and mild discomfort—a state with which most of us need to refamiliarize ourselves. Wait until hunger is an actual physical sensation, not just an emotional, mental, or spiritual craving.)

And when it comes to choosing the kinds of food we'll put in our mouths, many of us have become hooked on instant foods. What we see in an ad or smell as we pass a bakery or restaurant pulls at us. We have developed unhealthy addictions to what's fast and fake and fatty and full of additives. We have drowned out the voice of our internal regulator, which is always trying to lead us to nutritious choices.

We don't need to implant anything new into our wonderfully designed bodies. We need, instead, to strip away the distracting voices of this world that rush and tempt and accuse and confuse us. We need to sit still before the Lord and ask him to slow us down and teach us to listen to our bodies. He will give us the patience to allow the friendly growls of our stomachs to act as our dinner bells. He will free us to hear what foods our bodies are really asking for and give us the courage to respond.

—CDC

Prayer

Father, I thank you for my body, just as it is today. I know that I contain everything I need to begin to regulate my weight. I want to begin now, this minute, to live in real harmony with your perfect plan for me. You know what my ideal weight is, Lord, and you know the kinds and the amounts of food that I need to eat to reach that weight. Forgive me, Lord, for filling my body with unhealthy kinds and amounts of food. Forgive me for drowning out the natural cues that my body has been trying to give me over the years. Father, give me the patience now to wait for hunger as the cue for my meals. Help me to hear my body requesting the foods that it needs for health and wholeness. Help me to recognize the signal that my body is comfortably full, and give me the courage to stop eating then. I trust you and love you. In Jesus' name, Amen.

Scripture

God is working in you to help you want to do and be able to do what pleases him. (Philippians 2:13) (This is great news! Not only will he show us what to do, he will put within us a desire to do it and then give us strength to follow through!)

Food for Thought

We need to strip away the distracting voices of this world that rush and tempt and accuse and confuse us. We need to sit still before the Lord and ask him to slow us down and teach us to listen to our bodies. He will give us the patience to allow the friendly growls of our stomachs to act as our dinner bells. He will free us to hear what foods our bodies are really asking for and give us the courage to respond.

ASSIGNMENTS

1. Write the heading *Patience* at the top of the page. Look up these Scriptures; for future encouragement, write them in your notebook: Luke 21:19; Galatians 6:9; Psalm 37:7; James 1:3–4, 12; Psalm 40:1; Hebrews 10:35.

2. Consider: one reason diets don't work is that they are founded on negatives. Our minds and actions will never be motivated to act on such negatives as denying, depriving, or starving ourselves. Becoming faithfully fit draws and motivates us because it is founded on positives such as (1) living in joyful response to what God has given us, (2) doing kind and nourishing things for the marvelous temple he has created to house his Holy Spirit, (3) beginning to live in harmony with his perfect design for our lives—physically, spiritually, mentally, and emotionally.

3. The most successful plan to follow for healthy eating is one tailor-made for you. You must consider your lifestyle, body type, profession, and life goals. Spend some quiet time with the Lord this week, thinking and praying about these things. Ask him to help you design a perfect-for-you program: first, a program through which you can lose the amount you have decided on, and later, one by which you can live a serene and normal life.

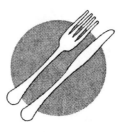

day 3: patience
a penchant for drama

I love before-and-after stories. I almost always stop to read the diet ads and gaze open-mouthed at photos of Clarissa Snodgrass, who has metamorphosed from a doughy wad of a person into a shapely shadow of her former self (usually with very little effort on her part).

That's the kind of story I thought at times I'd love to have: high voltage. How impressive to be able to say, "I used to weigh four hundred pounds, and then this miraculous thing occurred, and now I weigh 110, and I will forever!"

Why am I so drawn to the sagas of miracle weight loss? You might say I have a penchant for drama—high drama! Gradual changes have never made my heart go pitter-pat. I guess thirty-minute TV shows and thirty-second commercials have conditioned me to look for something flashy to happen in the bat of an eye.

Unfortunately, documenting my own real-life weight loss would take a lot more prime time than a thirty-minute sitcom (or even a six-week miniseries!). Over the years it has been a day-to-day, week-to-week, up-and-down journey.

I have vacillated from compulsive to contrite to complacent and back again many times over the past dozen or so years. I have fluctuated between several dress sizes, from slim to downright dumpy. I have tried stacks of quick-fix diets that appealed to my penchant for drama. I have experimented with countless numbers of weight control tricks and exercise gimmicks, but nothing about my eating really changed until I became willing to stop seeking the dramatic and acquire a desire for reality.

Today I have an earnest desire for what is available to me in Jesus Christ. Today I desire nothing less than a whole and healthy life. I long for a balanced view of all God's gifts in general, and of one in particular: food. I want to eat right and keep eating right. I want to stop overeating and stay stopped. I am entirely ready to let go of the fleeting lure of the dramatic. I desire the kind of sane and balanced life that is in line with what my God has for me today, for I know it will be his best! How could I desire more?

—LRB

Prayer

Father, your love is changing the world, and it is changing me. I desire to live in the reality of your love. Your story is one of grace and salvation. I lay my life and health and eating habits before you now. I pray that you will receive me in the fullness of your grace and in the glory of your victory. I desire what you have for me, and I long to honor you with everything I say and do and am. In the name of Jesus Christ I pray, Amen.

Scripture

Enjoy serving the Lord,
and he will give you what you want. (Psalm 37:4)

Food for Thought

Once you are willing to stop seeking quick-fix diets and weight control gimmicks, you'll be ready to adopt the sane and balanced lifestyle of eating and exercising that the Lord has in mind for you, the child he created, the child he loves.

ASSIGNMENTS

1. During your quiet time, ask God to show you where you have been in your patterns of eating, where you are now, and specifically where he wants you to go. (If you ask specifically, he will show you specifically.) Write out your insights.

2. Write your "before" story in the Journal section of your notebook. Then write a prayer that asks the Lord to help you follow his specific directions, which will lead you to your own positive "after" story. Describe the "after" story as you imagine it.

3. As you exercise remind yourself, "But we thank God! He gives us the victory through our Lord Jesus Christ" (1 Cor. 15:57).

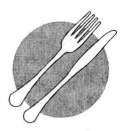

day 4: patience
one day at a time

When Jesus spoke the words "Don't be anxious about tomorrow" (Matt. 6:34 TLB), he was disclosing to us an amazing and life-changing secret: God will take care of our tomorrows as we learn to live this one day today.

We take every journey only one step at a time. Each person lives a lifetime only one day at a time. We live every day of our lifetimes only one moment at a time. How much more joy each of us would find available to us if we could really live as if we believed this truth.

This journey of change that we are taking together unfolds gradually. God works in our hearts and attitudes gradually. What we don't understand today will become clearer and clearer if we'll just keep on keeping on. I promise you that God does not disappoint. Many years ago my friend Lynn Keesecker wrote a wonderful song about God's faithfulness, and he called it "Promise Keeper." Now a worldwide ministry is known by that wonderful title. Our God really is a promise keeper who never fails us nor forsakes us. Oh, how each of us needs a deep belief in that reality!

So if you feel you're not getting there fast enough, don't speed up. Slow down! What's the rush? Stop pushing. If you have surrendered your life (and your eating behaviors) to God, then the process is working. He is at work on your behalf just as he promised he would be. If you are staying in his presence in prayer, then you are changing, whether you can see the changes right now or not.

I find that the Lord opens up new understanding and incorporates new changes only as I become ready to receive them. Just as elementary school teachers hold back certain lessons until they are convinced the children are ready, so does our heavenly Parent hold back lessons in our lives. Our job is to remain steadily on the journey. The changes will come. His timing is impeccable.

Many of us who have struggled with food issues (and I am no exception) tend to be perfectionists in one form or another. When you combine perfectionism with impatience (which tends to be another one of our common traits), you come up with a person who wants to be totally fixed, healed, skinny, and perfect right now. The anxiety those thoughts can stir up is something we do not need if we plan to stay on course.

One of my favorite slogans, which is said to have originated in Alcoholics Anonymous, is "Progress, Not Perfection." Just the fact that you are reading a book designed to help you is progress. So give yourself some credit, and relax. Perfection will come about in heaven in "the twinkling of an eye." When we see him, we will be like him. That's what Scripture tells us, and that's good news! In the meantime, the Lord is at work in our lives, one minute at a time. Let's give him some space to work!

—CDC

Prayer

Lord Jesus, I thank you that your timing is perfect in all things. And even though I cannot always feel or see it, Lord, I thank you that you are at work in my life right this minute. I release to you, Lord, my own plans and my own timetable. You are in control, and I trust you, in your way and in your time, to bring about your perfect will in my life. I surrender this day to you. Help me to live out each small moment, trusting your goodness.

Scripture

By your endurance you will gain your lives. (Luke 21:19 NASB)

Food for Thought

You'll find that the Lord opens up new understanding and incorporates changes in your life only as you become ready to receive them. Just as elementary school teachers hold back certain lessons until they are convinced the children are ready, so does our heavenly Parent hold back lessons in our lives. So stay steadily on the journey. The changes will come. His timing is impeccable.

ASSIGNMENTS

1. Find the joy in this day. In your Journal section, write a description of your life at this moment, focusing on the good aspects of your surroundings. Determine to move deliberately and thoughtfully through this day, without rushing.

2. During your quiet time this morning, take fifteen to twenty minutes just to sit and bask in God's love for you. You don't have to prove yourself to him. He knows all about you, and he loves you anyway. He likes you, too; as a matter of fact, he's crazy about you!

3. Concentrate on having an unrushed, peaceful attitude about everything you do today—even exercise. Enjoy even the calm and deliberate act of changing into your exercise clothing, and enter into your workout with enthusiasm and abandon. Forget about how it was yesterday or what's ahead tomorrow. Just enjoy moving your body today!

day 5: patience
leaving room for his best

At a dinner party recently, at the end of a delicious meal, our hostess brought out a beautiful platter of fruit for dessert. A woman sitting near me gazed sadly at the delectable array and moaned, "Oh no! I couldn't put one more thing in my body."

I must admit I identified with the overfed guest immediately. How many times have I been there, hating that stuffed feeling and wishing I had not given my appetite full rein?

There is much to be said for leaving room in our lives for something more. Stuffing ourselves with food is a pretty good metaphor for all the other ways we overstuff our lives—with too much busyness, too many meaningless activities, a clutter of surface relationships, and a tangle of material possessions.

When we satiate our physical appetites to the point of being stuffed, we are left feeling bloated, uncomfortable, and somehow still dissatisfied. We wish we had been more selective, more self-controlled. When we metaphorically stuff our lives with things and activities, we are left burned-out, exhausted, and dissatisfied—because we have left no room for the truly rewarding people and pursuits for which we should have saved time.

The growing incidence of bulimia (bingeing on food and

then "purging" with laxatives or induced vomiting) demonstrates how many young people are stuffing more these days and enjoying it less. A university in our area has even had to post signs in the women's bathrooms instructing the girls not to purge there—the high amount of stomach acid was affecting the plumbing!

I believe that stuffing ourselves is an activity born of fear. We fear that there will not be enough of what we need to satisfy us later on, so we decide to glut ourselves with what is available here and now. We also cram food in our mouths (and activities into our lives) as a way of anesthetizing ourselves from our true feelings. And it works—but only temporarily. And the consequence of our stuffing—besides fat and fatigue—is that we crowd out the good things God has in store for us.

Thinking about fullness and emptiness led me to the Bible, where I found a very interesting passage. Luke 1:53 says, "He has filled the hungry with good things and sent the rich away with nothing." This wording caused me to think that perhaps the rich people's lives are already full of what their money can buy—not only food, but possessions and activities as well. The poor people, on the other hand, are empty. They come in need, with space in their lives for the good things God is waiting to supply.

I am learning to look at hunger as a good, positive feeling—a sensation tinged with the excitement and anticipation of all that God, our Provider, has in store. He wants us to be hungry for his best. He wants us to live in patient, faithful anticipation, trusting him to fill our hungry lives with good things.

—CDC

Prayer

Lord God, I confess to you that I have frequently stuffed my body with more food than was healthy. I have stuffed my schedule with more activities and my closets with more possessions than I needed. I repent of the excesses in my life, and I confess the fear that has motivated my behavior. I turn to you now as my loving Provider, trusting you to supply my every need. Grant me the grace and the patience to choose the moderate path in the present moment, as I leave my future moments in your hands. In Jesus' name I pray, Amen.

Scripture

Why spend your money on food that doesn't give you strength? Why pay for groceries that do you no good? Listen and I'll tell you where to get good food that fattens up the soul! (Isaiah 55:2 TLB)

Food for Thought

God is our Provider. He wants us to be hungry for his best as we live in faithful anticipation, trusting him to fill our lives with good things.

ASSIGNMENTS

1. Too often we load up our foods with high-calorie dressings, gravies, and sauces. This week, concentrate on ordering and preparing foods without a lot of extras. God's best is *au naturel.*

2. We are to be filled with the character of God. Read Luke

1:46–55 (Mary's song of praise). In your Journal, list the qualities of God described in this beautiful passage.

3. Consider: when we stuff our bodies with food, we mistakenly believe that we are treating ourselves, when actually we are harming ourselves. As we trust God and seek more healthy ways of eating, we learn better how to judge exactly what our bodies need to function at their best. Then we choose to eat only these things, and only in moderate amounts.

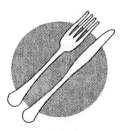

keeping on keeping on

Winston Churchill was once asked to deliver the commencement address at a school where he had been a student years before. The graduates and their families waited in great anticipation for the wise words of this elder statesman. Churchill stood, walked to the podium, looked out over his audience for a long moment, and began to speak.

"To you who are going out into the world today, I have three important things to say." The audience members leaned forward in their seats.

"Never give up!" he said. "Never give up! *Never* give up!" Winston Churchill sat down.

This oft-repeated anecdote is very applicable to us as we strive to change our eating habits. Perseverance is a key ingredient in success of every kind, and our challenge is no exception. Perseverance is a must as we allow the Lord to remold the attitudes and behaviors of a lifetime. In our struggle to conquer overeating, we must keep on keeping on.

I remember my favorite eighth-grade teacher's saying that often a person's tenacity determined his or her success. Many times the outstanding achiever is merely the person who did not quit on her dreams. There are so many things to dissuade us on the way. We must decide early in the journey that nothing will turn us back.

Our sons Curt and Andy both ran track in high school. Their championship coach, Jim Tate, believes that track is an excellent character builder, and Curt concurs with this assessment. He says that in his college career, it was track more than any other discipline that taught him to dig in and keep going.

In the New Testament, Paul often spoke of life as a race. He likened our need to hang in there to the discipline of a runner who never turns back. And he spoke of the need for perseverance as we go for the finish line: "I know that I have not yet reached that goal, but there is one thing I always do. Forgetting the past and straining toward what is ahead, I keep trying to reach the goal and get the prize for which God called me through Christ to the life above" (Phil. 3:13–14).

We need this kind of determination as we pursue the goal of living obediently before God in the areas of eating and exercise. There is no mystery to where we'll be if we give up now: right back where we started. We already know how that felt, and we didn't like it. That's why we started this journey in the first place.

Perhaps you were gung-ho in the beginning of your commitment, but lately you've felt your enthusiasm wane. If so, this is an excellent time to take steps to get recharged! The assignments for today offer some practical suggestions.

—CDC

Prayer

Father, I thank you for never quitting on us. You never swerve from your purposes, and you never change from age to age. I confess to you that I am in need of a touch from you. My strength runs out, and my determination sags at times. But you have boundless energy and power. I thank you that the very same power that raised Christ from the dead dwells in me because I believe in you. Help me to live out of that power. Keep me strong and on course. Revitalize my commitment. In Jesus' name, Amen.

Scripture

So let us run the race that is before us and never give up. We should remove from our lives anything that would get in the way and the sin that so easily holds us back. Let us look only to Jesus, the One who began our faith and who makes it perfect. He suffered death on the cross. But he accepted the shame as if it were nothing because of the joy that God put before him. And now he is sitting at the right side of God's throne. (Hebrews 12:1–2)

Food for Thought

I will keep my eyes on Jesus as I move toward my goal.

ASSIGNMENTS

1. Rewards are a tremendous motivator. Many rewards and benefits will be yours as a result of changed eating behavior. Make a list of these. Examples: (1) feeling better physically, (2) improved appearance, (3) increased self-esteem, and so on. Make your list very personal by including your own details. In addition to these intrinsic rewards, you may wish to schedule an external treat for yourself at the end of each week as a reward for perseverance. (No food rewards,

please!) Suggestions: a new scarf or earrings, a visit with someone you love, a trip to the library or to a museum, or a long-distance call. Write your schedule of rewards in the Goals section of your notebook.

2. If you're using the buddy system, call your buddy and share how you're feeling. Confide your need for support and prayer as you persevere toward your goals. If you don't have a buddy, make a point of talking to someone about how you feel. Don't try to be a Robinson Crusoe Christian or a Lone Ranger Reformer. We all need each other.

3. Get on your knees. Be real with God so he can be real to you. Tell him you need a fresh touch of enthusiasm. The word *enthusiasm* comes from the Greek words *en theos*, which literally mean "in God." Apart from him, our spirits fail us. But his Spirit never fails. In him, our engines get revved!

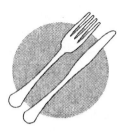

patience with our feelings

Jacque's house has termites, and is she mad! Just when she and Phillip were whittling their debts down to a manageable size, they are stuck with a nine-hundred-dollar bill just to repair the damages, not to mention the charge for a contract with an exterminator.

When Jacque found out, she called Phillip at work to tell him. He tried to cheer her up by saying, "Well, it could have been worse." But that didn't help her a bit.

"I know they could be worse, Phillip," she said. "But that doesn't change anything. Right now I'm just plain furious. I'm mad at myself for not getting the termite bond in the first place. I'm mad at the termites for making a meal out of our home. I'm even mad at God for thinking up termites in the first place. And I've got to go ahead and feel this anger, or it'll get buried inside of me and pop out later in the form of depression—which inevitably leads me to the cookie jar!"

Jacque fumed and fussed off and on for most of the morning. But by the time I talked to her this afternoon, she was feeling a lot better and even laughing a little bit about it. She said she remembered Corrie ten Boom's account in *The Hiding Place* of the fleas in the prison camp and how God used them for a blessing.

"I can't imagine how he'll use these dumb termites for a blessing," she chuckled. "But if he did it with fleas, I guess it's possible!"

Jacque is a very wise lady. She has learned to recognize and feel her feelings and express them appropriately. She doesn't try to leapfrog over them or deny their existence. She has the patience and faith to stop where she is and deal with them.

That doesn't mean she wallows around in them for months on end. But she doesn't ignore them or pretend they aren't there. She doesn't rush to cover them up with spiritual Band-Aids.

Jacque says she has learned to treat anger (and other negative feelings) as she might treat one of her children who needs to be taken seriously: she listens and responds appropriately. When she does, she finds the feeling is much more willing to run off and play in somebody else's yard!

Feelings that we don't experience and deal with honestly can gain a subtle kind of power over us. They frequently go underground and crop up in the form of inappropriate behavior that seems to come out of nowhere. We may cry for no reason or have unreasonable outbursts of temper. And if food happens to be our weakness, we may overeat!

That is definitely the case with me. Like Jacque, I have found that when I keep myself from facing my feelings and dealing with them on the spot, they almost always become subtle triggers for my compulsive eating. I'll find myself using a bout with food as a subconscious release for the emotions I have pushed down or denied. But once I slow down long enough to experience my feelings honestly and commit them to God, they no longer have the power to hurt me.

—CDC

Prayer

Lord, thank you for making us so wonderfully complex. Thank you for giving us minds and bodies and emotions and spirits. Lord, I know that you are not content to heal us in only one area of our lives; you long to make us whole (holy) in your sight. By the power of your Holy Spirit, help us to be aware of our feelings. Give us the patience and the courage to deal with them honestly so that they may gain no power over us. We surrender our whole selves to you—bodies, minds, emotions, and spirits—trusting you to lead us into wholeness of life. In Jesus' name, Amen.

Scripture

[The Lord] will bring to light the things that are now hidden in darkness, and will make known the secret purposes of people's hearts. (1 Corinthians 4:5)

Food for Thought

Feelings that we don't experience and deal with honestly can gain a subtle kind of power over us. They frequently go underground and crop up in the form of inappropriate behavior such as emotional outbursts or overeating. Far better to deal honestly with our emotions so that they may gain no power over us. Recognize them, express them, and surrender them to God.

ASSIGNMENTS

1. When you have been tempted to overeat, you may wish to go back and analyze in writing what you were feeling. Was some underlying emotion driving you? Were you angry

119

with yourself or someone else? Were you feeling guilty? Were you anxious over something, or fearful? Ask the Lord to help you untangle your feelings and face them. Respond appropriately. (Do you need to express your feelings to someone else, confess to God, ask for advice or prayer from a friend, take care of something you've been procrastinating about?) Take some action to deal with your feelings rather than eating to cover them up.

2. Consider: many of us have powerful food cues attached to childhood memories or feelings. Family reunions or visits from certain family members, certain holidays or traditions, or simply replays of mental tapes from our past may cause us to flash back to food-associated feelings that lead to overeating. (These memories can be positive or negative.) Learning to feel our feelings, deal with our emotions, and work on present-day relationships are steps that can keep us from the clutches of a "food flashback"!

3. This week, don't choose the handiest parking place. Consciously choose one that will cause you to do some extra walking in order to reach your destination. Those extra steps add up!

week five: choosing

choos•ing (chōōz´ in͡g), v. 1. to select in preference. 2. to decide or desire.

Aside from breathing, choosing may be the activity most common to human beings. Every day brings a series of choices. In some sense we may even view the primary function of human life as that of "chooser." The sum of our choices certainly determines to a large extent who and what we become.

It would seem that human beings, once educated as to what choices will prove to be in their best interest, would be able to choose wisely and well. Unfortunately, this is not always the case. Blame it on rebellion, human weakness, stubbornness, or original sin, but the fact remains: a large portion of the world's population goes through life making less-than-ideal choices day after day.

In the areas of eating and exercise, for instance, many of us have developed a pattern of destructive choosing. We have turned away from healthy, nourishing options (though we have known they were good for us) and have gone instead for harmful quantities and kinds of food coupled with a lack of exercise.

We will spend this week, therefore, considering this matter of choice. We will evaluate our own past choices and seek God's strength to reverse some of the negative trends we may discover. We can be sure that our recovery from destructive eating will come about as our choices begin to line up with God's will for our lives.

I Will Choose Your Way

So many things I need to learn,
So many different ways to turn
So many times I feel confused,
But in the end, my heart will choose.

Chorus:
I will choose your way
Every hour, every day;
Finding joy as I obey,
I will choose your way
I will choose your way
Every crossroad on the way
With a heart that's filled with praise
I will choose your way.

So many things I could believe
So many things unclear to me
But there's a simple truth I know
Of who I'll choose, and where I'll go.

Repeat chorus

Bridge:
You are always faithful, always true
You're the one I'll always choose.

Repeat chorus

—Claire Cloninger

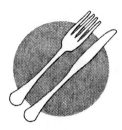

day 1: choosing
everyday choices

It's fine to talk in lofty terms about spiritual power. But one of the daily realities of our lives is this: three times a day—at least—we've got to have a face-to-face showdown with food. We've got to choose what to chew! God doesn't send an angel into the cafeteria line to take away all temptation. And for those of us with food issues, choosing can be stressful!

At times I have even entertained a notion that it would be nice if I didn't have to choose at all. It would be much easier on me if God would just take away that responsibility and make me do the healthy thing.

To reflect on the basics of human choice, however, is to see why that notion would go against the very grain of who God created us to be. The ability to choose is one of the ways he made us in his image: we are choosers as he is a chooser. Unlike any other created being, we have been granted the ability to consider thoughtfully and make conscious choices.

Rather than fearing, resenting, or shying away from choice, we should rather embrace the privilege thankfully. We can seek God's will in each small choice and receive his strength for making that choice wisely.

Am I saying that God cares whether we choose broccoli or

lima beans Friday at lunch? In a way, yes. I believe that the Lord cares about each decision we have to make, and that if we are tuned in to him and walking in the Spirit, he will give us guidance to choose well.

If you are currently on a nutrition or weight-loss program that outlines what you are to eat each day, pray over your list each morning. Ask God to strengthen you to make each small choice in accordance with your program.

If you are not on a specified diet but feel that it is time to begin changing your eating habits, God will help you choose the diet or eating program that is best and healthiest for you. You may even be considering counseling or a support group to help you with your eating problem. Put that decision before him too. Ask him to lead you to the right choice, and he will.

Still, we all know it is one thing to know which choice to make and quite another thing to be strong enough actually to make it. So here's the added benefit that makes all the difference: our God not only leads us to recognize the best choices for our lives (his will), he also provides us with the power we need for making those choices (his Holy Spirit). Philippians 2:13 makes this point: "God is working in you to help you want to do and be able to do what pleases him." Even when the right choice seems uncertain, we can rely on God's promise to be with us, guiding and strengthening us as we seek his will.

—CDC

Prayer

Lord God, thank you for giving me the privilege of making choices. I confess to you that I have made many wrong choices in the past. I need your help, your guidance, and your strength in my choosing. Help me to seek your will in every small choice, Father, and provide me with the inner strength to follow through on those choices as you reveal them to me. In Jesus' name, Amen.

Scripture
I will make you wise and show you where to go. I will guide you and watch over you. (Psalm 32:8)

Food for Thought
The Lord strengthens his children to make healthy and healing choices. It is his desire not only to give you the wisdom to know what is the best for you but to give you the strength to make that choice.

ASSIGNMENTS

1. If you have not already done so, ask the Lord to guide you in choosing (1) your own program of eating, and (2) your own regular regimen of exercise. Choose an eating and exercise program that offers variety and challenge but is also realistic. Take time choosing what is best suited for you.

2. Review your goals today. Have you by now set some small stepping-stone goals that lead to your major goals? Evaluate your progress on these. Beside each one write out the road-blocks that may be holding you back. Beside each of these roadblocks, list at least one method for overcoming or

removing that roadblock. (Example: Your roadblock may be "I find myself tasting the dishes I am cooking as I prepare the evening meal." Your method for overcoming that roadblock might be "I will fix myself a no-calorie drink to sip as I cook. I will take only one final taste before serving and adjust my seasoning at that point.")

3. Consider: choosing is a habit. We can change the habitual choices we make by always repeating alternative choices. Repetition makes a new groove in the brain through which our choices can travel. Don't be discouraged if you revert to old habits occasionally. Determine what your new course of action will be and continue to choose it until the new pattern begins to overcome the old.

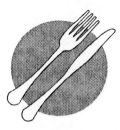

day 2: choosing
less is more

Several weeks ago my husband, Spike, clipped a cartoon out of *The New Yorker* that really hit my funny bone. A typical Thanksgiving-type cornucopia was pictured. But instead of bounteous amounts of fabulous food pouring forth from its opening, there were only a few carrots and celery stalks. The caption read, "Horn of Moderation."

Why is this so funny? I asked myself. The answer came immediately. Given the choice between a horn of plenty and a horn of moderation, you'd think anyone in her right mind would reach for the horn of plenty. Yet every day, three times a day, I am trying to choose moderation. No wonder the cartoon made me laugh. It was ridiculing my daily struggle.

It's a little uncomfortable to realize that we live in one of the only countries in the world where people have any choice at all in the matter of "too much," "too little," or "just right" (to paraphrase Goldilocks). Most places on the globe, people take what little food they can find and are thankful for what they get, however meager it may be. But we, as citizens of this affluent nation, have the luxury of choosing to eat sensibly or not.

Some years ago our friend Gerrit Gustaffson attended a huge world hunger conference in the Philippines. One of the speakers there defined a wealthy person according to world standards as "someone who can eat at his or her discretion." By this definition, most of us in this country are wealthy.

But does having the privilege and opportunity to choose mean that we should abuse our bodies by overeating? As Paul says in Romans, "God forbid!" God calls us to be stewards of his bounty. He has provided a horn of plenty to us as a nation and left the choice to us. Will we choose to stuff our faces with more than we need, starve ourselves by eating too little, or use his gifts wisely by choosing just the right amount and kind of foods to best nourish our bodies?

Choosing healthy foods in reasonable quantities is a way of saying "thank you" to our God who has provided us with all good things. By avoiding unhealthy extremes in our eating, we are honoring our bodies as temples of his Holy Spirit. Choosing to share what we have with others less fortunate than we are is another important way to show our gratitude for God's abundance.

—CDC

Prayer

Lord God, thank you for providing for our needs. Thank you for the plenty available to us in this nation. Let us never take for granted the privilege we have of choosing to eat wisely. Yet, Father, we know ourselves well enough to know that all too often we make unwise choices. We need you, O Lord. We need the strength and the guidance of your Holy Spirit to empower us to choose well. We confess to you the times that we have followed our sinful appetites and compulsions into disobedience.

We repent and turn back to you, trusting you to grant us for-giveness, redemption, and the power to live for you. In Jesus' name we pray, Amen.

Scripture
You know these things—now do them! That is the path of blessing. (John 13:17 TLB)

Food for Thought
Choosing to eat healthy foods in reasonable quantities is a way of saying "thank you" to our God who has provided us with all good things. By avoiding unhealthy extremes in our eating, we are honoring our bodies as temples of God's Holy Spirit.

ASSIGNMENTS

1. During your quiet time, ask the Lord to reveal to you some ways that you can be more moderate in your eating. Tell him that you wish to bring your eating in line with his perfect will for your life. Listen for his "still, small voice" by sitting quiet-ly and focusing your attention on him for ten uninterrupted minutes. You may wish to repeat the words *Your will, not mine* silently to yourself when your mind wanders. After ten min-utes, write in the Insights section of your notebook any ideas that may have come to you about eating moderately.

2. Get together with your prayer partner and brainstorm some ways you might share your plenty with less-fortunate people close to home or abroad. I'm sure there are charities that distribute food to the poor in your own town.

3. Consider: moderation can also be a good idea when it comes to exercise. Pushing too hard can result in injuries or simply lead to burnout. A great workout is one that is challenging enough to work up a good sweat but not so rigorous as to strain or injure. Walking is an excellent workout for most people for the simple reason that it can be challenging and rewarding without presenting many risks.

day 3: choosing
temple for a king

On a bluff overlooking the deep bend of a sand-bottomed Alabama river, we built a log cabin with our own hands. It is spare and simple and blends perfectly with the pines and junipers and river and sky—so perfectly that sometimes I think if God himself had built a cabin on this site, it would have been exactly like ours. We call this little outpost of heaven "Juniper Landing."

It is interesting to consider the symbolism in the Bible that compares our bodies to houses, temples, tents, and dwelling places. According to Holy Scripture, my body is the address where my spirit, mind, personality, and sense of humor reside.

When God the Father strung together the particular combination of genetic components that make up each person, he must certainly have had something special in mind. And just as our little cabin on the river harmonizes with its surroundings, the bodily temple that each of us is constructing should harmonize closely with what we perceive to be God's original blueprint and design for us.

Henry David Thoreau, the great writer and naturalist, once observed that "every man is the builder of a temple, called his body, to the God he worships, after a style purely his own . . . We are all sculptors and painters, and our material is our own flesh and blood and bones."[1]

More amazing than the fact that we make our homes in these flesh-and-bone dwelling places is the incredible reality that the day we receive and acknowledge Jesus Christ as Lord, he moves in to stay! If we let him, he even takes over as Master of the household and begins calling the shots on the construction and renovation that are constantly going on in this, his holy temple.

This perspective should vitally affect every choice we make regarding food and exercise. For incredibly, each thing we put on our plates becomes a building block in the house that Jesus Christ has chosen to call home. And strange as it seems, each hour of physical exercise we enter into strengthens his outer walls and beautifies his living room!

God takes the care and maintenance of his holy temple very seriously, and so must we! "Don't you know that you are God's temple and that God's Spirit lives in you? If anyone destroys God's temple, God will destroy that person, because God's temple is holy and you are that temple" (1 Cor. 3:16–17).

—CDC

Prayer

Lord, I am filled with wonder to think that you would make my body your dwelling place. As I remember this, help me to treat my body with more respect and honor. Remind me, when I am choosing what I will eat, that I am building and caring for your temple. Give me the clear vision and courage to choose the healthiest possible materials. In Jesus' name I pray, Amen.

Scripture

What common ground can idols hold with the temple of God? For we, remember, are ourselves temples of the living God, as God has said:

> I will dwell in them and walk in them:
> And I will be their God, and they shall be my people.
>
> (2 Corinthians 6:16 PHILLIPS)

Food for Thought

Your body is the temple of God's Holy Spirit. Think on that today as you select your food and exercise your body. You are a temple and God dwells in you. This is serious stuff. Have a little respect for that body of yours!

ASSIGNMENTS

1. Think of yourself as a dwelling place for God. Apart from choosing the food that best builds and maintains his temple, what other considerations might you have? In what ways could you make your life a more beautiful and comfortable place for him to live? What kinds of books or reading material are you bringing into his house? What kind of music? Are you providing times of rest and times of celebration in his home? Write down your ideas in the Journal section of your notebook.

2. You may have discovered that your temple has become like a squirrel cage of destructive habits, and that you have been

going round and round in the same negative ruts. Reading this book is part of your decision to change.

3. Think of God as an interior (and exterior) decorator. Consult with him about the ways he is remodeling this dwelling place, your body, where he resides. Draw up a maintenance plan to begin using when this program is over and your goals have been met. List specific steps you might take to continue the good work you have begun. Record these ideas in the Planning section of your notebook.

day 4: choosing
a better choice

My friend Richard has lost seventy-two pounds! It's incredible; he doesn't even look like the same person. A group of us went to lunch the other day, and no fewer than three people came up to him and marveled at the transformation.

"How did you do it, Richard?" they all wanted to know. He made lots of jokes such as "I starved myself for ten months." Later I had a chance to ask him in earnest. "No, really," I said. "How did you do it?"

"It was so simple," he answered. "Not easy, mind you, but simple."

"Well?" I persisted. "Don't keep me in suspense. I'm writing a book about these things, and my readers await your answer."

"A better choice," he said mysteriously. "I used the principle of 'the better choice.'"

"You'll have to expand on that, Richard," I said. And he did.

"My day is always full of little decisions and mini-crossroads," he explained. "When I come to one, I just ask myself a simple question: what is the better choice? Then I choose it. That's it."

"That's it?" I said, disappointed.

"That's it," he repeated.

"Well, give me some examples," I urged.

"Okay," he continued. "I'm in a restaurant. I open the menu. Am I going to order the grilled chicken or the barbecued ribs? Obviously, the grilled chicken is the better choice. I choose it. Or it's Saturday morning. I have two hours before I'm supposed to pick up my daughters to take them shopping. Am I going to have a lazy soak in the tub, two cups of coffee, and a long session with the daily paper? Or am I going to have a brisk two-mile walk, a hot but hurried shower, and a glance at the headlines? Because I know I need the exercise, I opt to fit in the walk.

"Or I'm in the grocery store, loading up my cart for the week ahead. I linger for a moment over the picnic ham, but I notice right next to it a frozen turkey breast. I reach for the turkey.

"It's no big mystery. It's just a way of looking at things that has become a habit. I've even begun to think of it as a game. It works."

Since that conversation, I've used Richard's principle of "the better choice" in my own life and found it to be amazingly helpful. In fact, the more I've thought about it, the more it seems to me that we could play much of the game of life according to this simple principle. With Jesus Christ as our Guide, helping us choose wisely at every small crossroads, how simple our daily journey becomes! (Not easy, but simple.)

—CDC

Prayer

Lord Jesus Christ, I thank you for walking through this world before us, and that we can trust you to be our guide at every crossroads. Help us, Lord, to see each choice in the light of your wisdom. Empower us to choose as you would choose. Be so present and real in every part of our lives that your choices become second nature to us. We pray in your precious name, Amen.

Scripture

I call heaven and earth to witness against you that today I have set before you life or death, blessing or curse. Oh, that you would choose life; that you and your children might live! Choose to love the Lord your God and to obey him and to cling to him, for he is your life and the length of your days. (Deuteronomy 30:19–20 TLB)

Food for Thought

Think about this each time you have a simple choice to make today: *Jesus Christ dwells within me. He will help me make the best possible choice here at this small crossroads.*

ASSIGNMENTS

1. Take time now to go over your commitments and plans for the days ahead. Put a star beside each commitment that may require you to make a choice. (Examples: grocery shopping, lunch with Susie, dinner party at the Swensons'.) Then cover each of these commitments with prayer, asking the Lord ahead of time to give you the grace to recognize each small crossroads in your week and to provide you with the wisdom to make the better choice.

2. You are affected positively or negatively not only by what you choose to eat, but by the people with whom you choose to spend time. Consider the people who make you feel positive and hopeful as opposed to those who make you feel inferior and discouraged. By choosing to spend a good part of your time with those who believe in and encourage you, you are being kind to yourself and enhancing your program of reform and recovery. Whenever there is a choice to be made, surround yourself with faith-filled, positive friends.

day 5: choosing
facing down temptation

I have a real ambivalence about holidays. On one hand, I am childlike in my joy over angels and shepherds, pilgrims and turkeys, flags and fireworks. On the other hand, I tend to go through every holiday season with the mind-set of running a gauntlet. On all sides I see lurking obstacles and perilous pitfalls waiting to sabotage my efforts to eat sensibly. Cakes and pies and turkey and dressing are waiting at every turn to trip me up.

Sometimes I get so frustrated with my susceptibility to temptation. I cry out with David, "How long, O Lord?" I've been fighting these same enemies all my adult life. What's wrong with me? Shouldn't I be beyond tempting by now?

The answer to that last question is no. Jesus Christ himself was never beyond the beckoning of various temptations as long as he was walking around in his "man suit." And neither are we. Temptation is part of the package we call "humanity," and the sooner you and I can recognize that fact as a given, the closer we will be to overcoming on a regular basis.

This morning in my quiet time, I took a look at the two major temptation passages in the Bible: Adam and Eve's ordeal in Genesis 3, and Jesus' wilderness experience in Luke 4. The temptations themselves were very similar; the outcomes radically different.

I found it very interesting and telling to realize that both temptations were initiated by an offer of something to eat. The serpent held out a luscious piece of fruit to Eve, and Satan offered to turn a stone into a loaf of fresh-baked bread for Jesus. Surely this must at least say to those of us who struggle with food that we are not weird or weak or terribly unusual. The physical appetite is Satan's natural first front of attack.

It's also obvious that each of these temptations had a deeper level of significance than mere calories. Satan in both cases was using food as a lure. He was attempting to coax God's children out from under God's authority by getting them to act independently. Isn't this also the core issue we are facing when we choose to abandon God's path of health and wholeness by overeating?

Of course, the most telling aspect of each temptation story is its outcome. Adam and Eve, by yielding, were forced into a place of anxiety and shame. Jesus, by resisting, was comforted and empowered for the difficult days ahead. In my own eating, yielding to temptation generally produces Adam-and-Eve results for me: rationalizing, hiding, self-condemnation, and estrangement. But I find that when I use God's power to resist temptation, I am given more power to resist future temptations, just as Jesus was in the wilderness!

—CDC

Prayer

Father, I thank you for my temptations, for they cause me to rely on you. I thank you that Jesus was tempted as we are, though he never yielded to his temptations. As you continue to form me into the image of him, help me to face my own temptations without giving in to them. Give me strength in the time of trial. Teach me more and more to rely on the power of your indwelling Spirit. In Jesus' name, Amen.

Scripture

And now [Jesus] can help those who are tempted, because he himself suffered and was tempted. (Hebrews 2:18)

Food for Thought

Jesus was never above being tempted while he was here on earth, and neither are we. Temptation is part of the human package. Because he has been tempted, he is able to help those of us who are tempted.

ASSIGNMENTS

1. Think about situations in which you are frequently tempted to overeat (times of day, events, situations, emotions). How can you begin to access God's power during these times in order to resist temptation more consistently? Write your ideas in the Journal section of your notebook.

2. Write on a piece of paper the following scriptures: Hebrews 2:18, 1 Corinthians 10:13, and Matthew 6:13. Tape these to the cabinets that hold those temptation foods, as well as to your refrigerator. You may even wish to tape one to your TV, if you tend to eat in front of it.

3. Review your goals. In what ways has temptation been sabotaging one or more of your goals? Construct a plan of action for standing against that temptation and record your plan in your notebook.

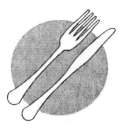

day 6: choosing
food as a substitute

just had a call from a friend who sounded upset. Her sales-man husband was out of town, she was stuck at home with three preschoolers, and she had just finished a heated argument with her sister-in-law (who gets on her nerves anyway). The result: my friend had dealt with her jangled nerves by consuming most of a half-gallon carton of rocky road ice cream and was now being consumed herself . . . by guilt.

How many of us have been in a stressful situation and reached for the ice cream? It's a pretty common scenario for overeaters. In fact, many of us have learned to use food to com-bat everything but what it was designed for—hunger. We reach for food when we're blue or angry or anxious or bored. We use food to punish ourselves or to reward ourselves. We use it for companionship, consolation, or celebration. We have turned to food for the comfort that can come only from God himself.

I have come to see this tendency in myself as a very subtle form of idolatry. When I allow my daily stresses to drive me to the refrigerator rather than to God, I have in some sense made food my god. I am like the people the apostle Paul described in Philippians 3:19 as "heading for utter destruction—their god is their own appetite" (PHILLIPS).

My friend realized, as she reflected on her afternoon, that her binge had been motivated by a spiritual hunger—one that no amount of ice cream could ever have satisfied. The emptiness she experienced had been triggered by feelings of loneliness (for her husband), anger (toward her sister-in-law), and guilt (over letting her temper get the best of her). Her real need was not for ice cream, but for forgiveness, reconciliation, and unconditional acceptance. Sadly she admitted that not only had the ice cream failed to meet her need, it had also distracted her from seeking God when she needed him most.

With God's help, we can begin to understand the hunger that drives us to overeat. Then we can choose instead to reach for his love that satisfies our real hunger.

—CDC

Prayer
Father, I ask you to forgive me for the times I have used food for a substitute god in my life.(Name specific times, if you can think of any.) Help me, Lord, to forgive myself. I release into your hands all feelings of guilt and shame, and I receive your forgiveness. I ask you now, Father, to help me replace my habit of reaching for food with the habit of reaching out to you. Give me strength and courage as I seek to change, and patience to continue this walk with you. In Jesus' strong name I pray, Amen.

Scripture
I am the Lord your God, who brought you out of the land . . . where you were slaves. You must not have any other gods except me. You must not make for yourselves an idol that looks like

anything in the sky above or on the earth below or in the water below the land. You must not worship or serve any idol, because I, the Lord your God, am a jealous God. (Exodus 20:2–5)

Food for Thought

When we allow the stress and struggles of daily life to drive us to food rather than to God, we are allowing food to become an idol in our lives.

ASSIGNMENTS

1. Prayerfully consider the circumstances that lead you to overeat: what, where, how, why, with whom, and how you felt. After a slip, make a point of writing it down in the Journal section of your notebook. (For example, you might write: "I had an argument with Lucy. Was very upset. Came home alone and ate two bowls of ice cream, standing up, rapidly. Felt better while eating but disgusted with myself afterward.") Ask the Lord to begin to reveal what motivates your negative eating behavior, and surrender these things to him to change.

2. I hope you are experiencing the blessings and the benefits of a daily quiet time by now. Ask God to give you a real hunger for that time you spend with him. Ask him to make it a choice of your heart, not an "ought to." Go to that appointment with him just as you would go to a special getaway with your best friend or your spouse.

3. Here's my number-one secret to exercise: just do it! I was a runner for eighteen enjoyable years. Though I choose now to walk, I've maintained the positive addiction to early morning exercise. I know its benefits, and I rarely miss. But that doesn't mean I always feel like going out. In my running days, I posted a small note to myself on the bathroom mirror that always helped get me into an exercise mode. It said simply: "Put your foot in the road!" I still make a habit of getting dressed and out the door before I can put up a mental argument.

day 7: choosing
he prepares a table

If I had to decide on my choice for the number-one psalm in King David's all-time Hit Parade, it would have to be the Twenty-third. I have loved this passage since childhood, and over the years I have probably spent as much time meditating on it as on any other passage of Scripture.

This morning as I was exercising, walking up and down on the wooded trail that leads to our cabin, I let those treasured lines roll around in my spirit again, and I got a fresh blessing. One line I had never particularly thought about before really stood out: "You prepare a meal for me / in front of my enemies" (v. 5).

What an incredible idea—that the King of kings and Lord of lords would stop at mealtime to fix lunch for me! As I marveled at that notion, I was reminded of the incident in the twenty-first chapter of John's gospel when Peter and the disciples returned from fishing and the resurrected Christ insisted on preparing breakfast for them from their catch. It would definitely be in character for him to prepare a table for me. Jesus—always the servant!

Suppose he were here today fixing our lunch. What would he choose to serve us? Knowing him to be the giver of good and perfect gifts, I'd guess it would be something simple and beautiful and nourishing.

"You prepare a table before me in the presence of my enemies" (NIV). Just who are my enemies when it comes to eating wisely and well? They are the ideas and emotions that cause me to lose my spiritual footing and make harmful choices. They are hurry and confusion, low self-esteem, depression, and the twin enemies self-pity and self-indulgence.

When Jesus prepares his table for me, he tells my enemies to stand back. They cannot touch me when he is in control. They cannot rush me or discourage me or tempt me into making a destructive choice. All of their clamoring is quieted in his presence. He spreads a beautiful cloth, sets the table with fine utensils, and places before me food that he knows will make me strong and healthy. Jesus Christ is the Host, and my enemies must sit uninvited outside his banquet!

—CDC

Prayer

Lord, I thank you for this beautiful picture you have given me from the Twenty-third Psalm. Thank you for promising to prepare a table for me in the presence of my enemies. As I prepare my meals today, may I remember that this is your table and that you are in control. Thank you for revealing to me that my enemies are not invited to your table. Quiet their clamoring voices so that I may eat the kind of food that is pleasing to you. May I make choices that are in perfect accord with the healthy, nourishing banquet you are inviting me to attend. Thank you for being my Host. Amen.

Scripture

Spend some time this week meditating on the beautiful words of the Twenty-third Psalm. Thank the Lord for being your Shepherd and Provider.

Food for Thought

Every meal we eat is a gift of heaven, and the Lord is our Host.

ASSIGNMENTS

1. Read John 21:1–14. Place yourself in the scene with the disciples. What are your feelings? What is surprising about this account? Where is the good news for you? Write your responses in the Journal section of your notebook.

2. Find at least one meal this week that you can eat alone. Set a place for the Lord and imagine that he is there with you sharing your table, your meal, and your thoughts. He is, you know!

3. Remove the words *should* and *ought* from your vocabulary when speaking about exercise. Even if you don't fully mean it yet, experiment with saying the following to yourself and/or others:

    *   "I'm looking forward to my workout this afternoon."
    *   "Nothing makes me feel quite as good as my morning walk."
    *   "I can feel my body thanking me every time I exercise."

Positive expressions like these will actually heighten your enjoyment of your workout. And before long, you'll really mean what you say!

week six: attitudes and disciplines

at•ti•tude (at´ i to͞od), n. 1. manner, feeling, etc., toward a person or thing. 2. posture expressive of an action, emotion, etc.

dis•ci•pline (dis´ ə plin), n. 1. training to act in accordance with rules. 2. instruction designed to train to proper conduct or action. 3. a system of order.

The final week of *Faithfully Fit* focuses on those attitudes and disciplines that can move us dramatically toward our goals. As we begin to build these qualities and practices into our daily lives, we find ourselves able to overcome in more areas than eating.

Though the daily meditations this week vary widely—covering such subjects as integrity, honesty, acceptance, planning, responsibility, fasting, self-control, and organization—each offers an avenue of help and hope to the overcomer by strengthening resolve and building character. We pray that these will become the tools that help keep you on course in the months ahead. With God's help they will become more and more a part of who you are in him. Our prayers are with you as you begin the last week of this program and the first week of a lifetime of victorious overcoming!

You In Me

In all I say and all I do,
In every view and attitude,
In every thought and every mood,
Let it be you in me.

Your love's invading all my days
And changing me so many ways,
Amazing joy, outpouring praise
That come from you in me.

Chorus:
You in me—not just me alone,
Oh what joy, joy that I've never known,
And Lord, you give me eyes to see
The way that I was meant to be
Oh Jesus, what a mystery
This love that's you in me.

And now I've got to praise your name,
Because you've broken every chain
Till love and love alone remains,
The love that's you in me.

Repeat chorus

Bridge:
Now everything is possible
Because you dwell within,
And every day it's more amazing
'Cause every day I see again . . .

Repeat chorus

—Claire Cloninger

day 1: attitudes and disciplines
what shapes you?

Laura's husband, John, doesn't like congealed salad. Doesn't trust it. "It's not only the unnatural color," he says, only partly in jest. "It's that I can't feel really comfortable about anything that takes the shape of whatever it's poured into. It's so . . . so devious!"

I know people who take the shape of whatever situation in which they find themselves. I've even been that way at times. Maybe you have too.

Part of honesty is knowing who we are and what we believe in regardless of the different kinds of situations in which we find ourselves. It's being who we are, not what others expect us to be. It's understanding the genetic determination of our own bodies and pursuing ideal fitness for ourselves based on that understanding. It is developing our own signature style of dressing rather than trying to be a clone of some emaciated body in a magazine ad.

If you're trying to look like a five-foot-eight fashion model and you're only five-two, you're obviously going against the grain of your own design. Our friend Maggie jokes about her short legs, saying that she and her siblings are the only people she knows whose legs are so short they don't even go all the way up to their fannies! Short legs are a genetic fact in her family of origin, and she is totally comfortable with that. Maggie is one of the most attractive women I know, with a style that is totally her own. She wouldn't dream of trying to imitate anyone else.

Understanding our own genetic determination means learning to be the best we can be within the limits of what God designed. There are certain things about our bodies that no amount of exercise will change. Jesus reminds us in the Sermon on the Mount that no amount of worry, struggle, or striving will "add one cubit to [our] stature" (Matt. 6:27 NKJV). Some things about us are just plain predetermined.

This doesn't mean that we must resign ourselves to being plump dumplings just because we had a pudgy mother or grandmother. My grandmother was quite stout, which was not uncommon for older women in her day. My mother, on the other hand, loves pretty clothes and is very health-conscious. She decided in the early years of her marriage that keeping her figure was worth the effort. Mama has always eaten wisely and exercised regularly, and at every age and stage of her life she has looked trim and beautiful.

The most important thing for us to know on this journey toward healthy eating is that God has a special design for each life. And as believers we are to be taking the shape of that perfect design rather than allowing the world to redesign us. Lest we become like congealed salads, we had best heed the words of the apostle Paul to the Christians at Rome: "Don't let the world around you squeeze you into its own mould, but let God remake you so that your whole attitude of mind is changed. Thus you will prove in practice that the will of God is good, acceptable to him and perfect" (Rom. 12:2 PHILLIPS).

—CDC

Prayer

Father, I thank you for designing me just as you did. I am thankful for the special plan you have for me. I want to cooperate with that plan in my life—in the way I eat and exercise, and in all of my decisions. Help me to be at peace with myself, not constantly striving to be something I am not. Give me the power to be the best I can be. Continue to reveal to me the ways that I can walk closer to your purposes in my daily life. In Jesus' name, Amen.

Scripture

> You made my whole being;
> you formed me in my mother's body. . . .
> You saw my bones being formed
> as I took shape in my mother's body.
> When I was put together there,
> you saw my body as it was formed. (Psalm 139:13, 15–16)

Food for Thought

Understanding our own genetic determination means learning to be the best that we can be within the limits of what God designed.

ASSIGNMENTS

1. In the Journal section of your notebook, list your physical characteristics that are genetic and unchangeable (short of major surgery). Examples might be your height, your bone structure, the length of your limbs, and so on. Now list your physical characteristics that can be improved by proper nutrition and exercise. Some examples are: your weight, your muscle tone, your measurements, and your skin tone.

2. Consider some specific benefits of moving your body (exercise): a brisk twenty-minute hike around the block burns off fifty calories just like that! Or if the weather's been bad, try stair climbing. It takes care of excess pounds to the tune of ten calories a minute! Now move it!

3. Reexamine your goals to make sure they are realistic and in harmony with your basic design. Really beautiful people are at peace with their body types and don't fight against them.

day 2: attitudes and disciplines
avoiding pitfalls

The girl was sixteen, petite, lovely, and a cocaine addict, recovering from an eighteen-month habitual pattern of drug use. Seated around her in her aftercare group were supportive counselors and fellow recovering addicts.

"Tomorrow is my first day back at school since I quit the drugs," she began in a trembling voice. "I'm scared to death. I'm afraid of seeing all the people I used with, and I'm afraid of seeing the ones who looked down on me for being a user. I'm afraid I won't have anyone to talk to. I'm afraid I won't be able to do the work. I'm afraid I'll use again. Let's face it—I'm afraid of everything!"

Gently, deliberately, her support group began to help her formulate a plan of reentry, a plan to help her face the temptations and avoid the pitfalls of this new situation. They gave her phone numbers of supportive people to call if she got in trouble. They listed names of people at the school (including a counselor) to contact right away. They asked her to think through potentially stressful situations ahead of time. And people in the group who had been through the same type of situation in their own recovery shared helpful and encouraging advice. Gradually an expression of hope and confidence replaced her look of terror.

What does this scenario have to do with our struggle to overcome overeating? Every new day we, too, are walking into situations fraught with temptations and pitfalls. What steps can we take ahead of time to prepare ourselves for those temptations so that we can stay on track with our own recovery from overeating?

Unlike the drug addict who realizes he or she must totally walk away from all narcotics, we who struggle with our eating behaviors cannot give up eating entirely, for obvious reasons. Our struggle is more subtle than that.

What we can and must do is honestly assess what our danger or trigger foods are. (That's easy for me. Mine are sweets and desserts. My husband, on the other hand, is pretty good at walking away from cheesecake, but he has a weakness for starches and salty snack foods.) Whatever your weakness is, it's a good idea to keep those food items out of your house altogether when you're changing your eating habits. If they are not there, you can't eat them—at least not without some effort! Anytime I find myself putting cookies or ice cream into my grocery cart, I know what's going on: I'm setting myself up for a fall. And with God's help, I stop myself.

Part of our journey toward eating sanely is learning to think through our weaknesses and temptations ahead of time rather than being caught off guard by them. With God's guidance and help, we can plan ahead and avoid the pitfalls.

—CDC

Prayer

Lord Jesus, as I think through the potential temptations of this day, help me to plan realistic ways to head them off. Give me the strength to remove from my environment any and all things that would be a stumbling block to my eating program. Help me not to fear my weakness but to trust your overcoming power in me. I thank you, Lord, for these places and times of testing that help me grow stronger in you. Amen.

Scripture:
But clothe yourself with the Lord Jesus Christ (the Messiah) and make no provision for [indulging] the flesh [put a stop to thinking about the evil cravings of your physical nature] to [gratify its] desires (lusts). (Romans 13:14 AMPLIFIED) (The key to this verse is "make no provision.")

Food for Thought
God has promised to help us when we are tempted. Consider this verse from 1 Corinthians: "The only temptation that has come to you is that which everyone has. But you can trust God, who will not permit you to be tempted more than you can stand. But when you are tempted, he will also give you a way to escape so that you will be able to stand it" (10:13).

ASSIGNMENTS

1. Think through the actual situations in your week that may prove stressful. (Are you going to a party where snacks, sweets, or other tempting foods may be served? Are you going out to eat with friends where you may be tempted to loosen your resolve? Are you going grocery shopping?) Ask

the Lord to guide you. Then, in the Planning section of your notebook, write out ways that will help you overcome in each of these situations.

2. Go through your kitchen and rid your cabinets and refrigerator of high-temptation foods (chips, candy, whatever tempts you). If you feel you must keep some of these on hand for your children or spouse, or if your roommate is not sympathetic to your new program, buy some plastic storage boxes, seal these temptations away from your first grasp, and put them on a high shelf or at the far back of a cabinet. They'll still be there, but you'll be surprised how just having them out of sight will help you resist.

3. If you are feeling weak as you consider the temptations at hand, praise God! Remember, God loves to be strong in weak people! Read 2 Corinthians 12:9 and paraphrase it in your Journal. Personalize it. Thank God for it!

day 3: attitudes and disciplines
avoiding avoiding

This is a rainy Wednesday afternoon, and my mind keeps returning to the contents of my refrigerator. I'm restless and distracted, and I feel as if a little food might be the answer. Wrong.

By now I am very familiar with these restless symptoms, and I know how to interpret them. Want to know what's really wrong? I'm avoiding something unpleasant. I'm procrastinating again. For three days I have been aware of a need to confront a business associate, but I dread the confrontation. Subconsciously I know that if I can have a good old-fashioned food binge, I'll feel bad enough about that to distract me from my primary problem. That way I can put off dealing with it a little longer.

Another lie I will sometimes tell myself is that I need extra food to build myself up for the difficult task at hand (the one I've been avoiding). The truth is that excess food bogs me down rather than revs me up. Stuffing my face may produce a temporary high, but an inevitable letdown follows once I realize what I have done. "A short-term euphoria is not worth the long-term anguish which inevitably follows loss of control."[1]

Anytime we are preoccupied with thoughts of food and eating, we should stop and take a serious inventory. What are we avoiding dealing with in the present? What is troubling us that

we would feel better putting behind us? We can ask the Lord to
show us the real cause of our restless desire to eat and then pray
about the best way to deal with it. We can ask him to reveal to us
his perfect will in the situation. If it's courage we need, or emotional energy, we can ask him to supply that. He can. He will.

One thing is certain: putting off dealing with a problem
does not make the problem disappear. And though compulsive
overeating may distract us temporarily, in the long run it only
serves to produce a secondary reason for feeling uncomfortable
and guilty.

Learning to face problems head-on now, with honesty and
courage, is taking an important step toward changing unhealthy
eating behaviors. Taking care of the business at hand, whatever
it may be, is a way of clearing the emotional decks for the devel-
opment of new and positive attitudes toward food and eating.

—CDC

Prayer

Lord Jesus, I confess the cowardice, fear, and laziness that keep
me from dealing with my problems promptly and honestly.
Lord, I know that you desire for me to be free of the nagging
clutter of unresolved conflicts. Father, I lift to you specifically
the thing(s) which concerns me now. (Here name the specific
area(s) and describe why they are hard for you to deal with.)
Lord, you know the person or people involved and the best way
to deal with this situation. I confess to you now any and all sinful attitudes I may be holding regarding this situation. (Here be
very specific about any dishonesty, fear, greed, resentment,

anger, or other negative attitudes you may be harboring.) Lord, I desire to clear the decks on this situation rather than distract myself from dealing with it by eating. Give me the courage and honesty I need to do what is required of me as your child. I praise you for your tender guidance and love as I seek to do your will. In Jesus' name I pray, Amen.

Scripture

Use every chance you have for doing good, because these are evil times. So do not be foolish but learn what the Lord wants you to do. (Ephesians 5:16–17)

Food for Thought

Anytime we are preoccupied with thoughts of food and eating, we should stop and take a serious inventory. Are we avoiding dealing with something? We can ask the Lord to show us the real cause of our restless desire to eat and then pray about the best way to deal with it.

ASSIGNMENTS

1. Write out the particulars of any situation that you have been avoiding. Be specific, just as you were in your prayer. After meditating on what you feel God is saying to you, write out what you feel to be his will for you in the situation. Write a target date for dealing with it. Make sure that the date you select is very soon. (Note: there may be more than one phase to what you need to do. Break your assignment into parts, if necessary.)

2. Now, begin to carry out your plan!

3. Many of us procrastinate about exercising. One way to combat that tendency is to have everything ready and waiting for your daily workout. I keep a basket in the bottom of our coat closet. In it are my workout clothes and shoes, a jump rope, two exercise videos, and a portable CD player with several up-tempo CDs. Though most mornings I walk for my exercise, I have my "exercise basket" always on the ready in case of rain, or in case I feel bored with my usual routine. Having them always available gives me no excuse for putting off the workout!

day 4: attitudes and disciplines
fasting as a tool

Though Scripture is full of spiritual imperatives urging the follower of God to fast regularly, until recently I had always tended to think of fasting as an extreme—something for monks and other fanatical people. Then the other day as I was reading the Sermon on the Mount for the many-eth time, I saw something new in Jesus' words about fasting.

It was in the part of the sermon where Jesus is instructing us on how to walk in the Way. He prefaces his instructions with the words "*when* you pray" and "*when* you give" and "*when* you fast." He does not say "if" you do these things, but "when." The follower of Christ is not presented with an option as to whether he will follow these three important disciplines. Jesus is taking it for granted that those who follow him *will* pray, give, and fast.

It struck me as significant that Jesus gave fasting the same weight of importance as praying and giving, two Christian virtues that no theologian would question. Yet many Christians (like me) who wouldn't dream of trying to walk the Christian journey without praying and giving have tended to see fasting as an outdated discipline, not relevant to the modern believer.

What current relevance does fasting have to us as believers in general and, more specifically, as believers who are seeking to restructure our eating habits? Fasting can be a tool to remind us that food is not to be our comfort. God is our comfort. Food will not bring us true peace when we are anxious. Only the Prince of Peace will do that. The bottom line is that Jesus is our Bread: the one who feeds us, the one who fills us.

Fasting can be an effective reminder of this truth. A weekly fast of one day gives my body a twenty-four-hour rest from consuming. It provides my spirit with a reminder that God is my comfort, my hope, and my strength.

To begin fasting regularly, seeking the Lord first is about the best way to begin. He may lead you to begin small, fasting only during breakfast and lunch one day a week, drinking plenty of juice and water. After you have established this partial fast as a regular part of your physical and spiritual life, he may lead you to move into fasting all three meals on your day of discipline.

Prayerfully entering into this scriptural discipline provides the Lord an opportunity to empty us of the fullness of this world so that he can fill us with the fullness of his kingdom. When we come to see fasting as God's provision for our well-being, we will be able to accept it gratefully as a gift from his hands.

—LRB

Prayer

Father, thank you for providing for my physical, mental, emotional, and spiritual needs. Thank you for the discipline of fasting and for all of the benefits available to me through it. I ask you, Lord, to direct me personally as to how I should begin to acquire this discipline in my own walk with you. Grant me the grace and the power I will need to follow through. I long to be emptied of the fullness of this world and filled instead with the fullness of your kingdom. In Jesus' name I pray, Amen.

Scripture

Then Jesus said, "I am the bread that gives life. Whoever comes to me will never be hungry, and whoever believes in me will never be thirsty." (John 6:35)

Food for Thought

A weekly fast of one day gives my body a twenty-four-hour rest from consuming. It provides my spirit with a reminder that God is my comfort, my hope, and my strength.

ASSIGNMENTS

1. Read Isaiah 58 and reflect on the heart attitude God desires of us when we fast. Describe it in the Journal section of your notebook.

2. Look through your calendar and obligations. Choose a day during which you can realistically plan to fast. Set that day aside and begin now to pray for the power you will need to follow through. (Note: you may wish to get a doctor's approval before beginning.)

3. Carry out your plan by fasting one day. Exercise lightly or not at all, and give your body a period of rest during the day.

Allow the hunger you are experiencing to draw your spiritual focus to the Lord. Listen to what he is saying to you during this special time. We are often able to hear him more clearly when we have disciplined ourselves to turn away from food and toward him only.

day 5: attitudes and disciplines
other rewards and consolations

My friend Betty was winning a courageous and difficult struggle to quit smoking except for one special time of day. After dinner, when the dishes were washed and the children were busy with homework, how she craved that last cigarette of the evening—the one she had thought of as a reward for a hard day's work.

One evening, as Betty prayed about her problem, the Lord gave her this answer. "Tonight let me be your after-dinner reward." And so that night, instead of settling down with a cigarette, Betty settled down with a good book—*the* Good Book, in fact! In less than a week of substituting Bible reading for smoking, she began to feel the craving weaken, and eventually it disappeared.

Many of us have developed eating habits much like Betty's smoking habit. We have created patterns of using certain foods at certain times of day as she used her cigarettes—for rewards or consolation prizes. We may be hooked on the idea that a meal is not complete without a dessert, for instance. Or maybe we have conditioned ourselves to come in from work and head straight for the refrigerator for a snack. Or our habit may be to indulge in a bedtime snack, even though we know those late-night calories are the hardest ones to shed.

Changing our eating behaviors is very difficult, but change is easier when we learn to substitute a positive activity for a negative one. It also helps to remember that overeating itself is often a substitute activity for what we're really craving—love and companionship. If we can take steps to fill the real longings in our lives, we won't have to keep stuffing ourselves with food to fill up the emptiness.

Here is a suggested list of "alternative" activities you may wish to try when you are tempted to eat:

- Keep a list of friends you've been meaning to touch base with and make a call instead of taking a bite! Keep the phone number of a special supportive friend handy and give her an SOS call when you're tempted to overeat.

- Put together a list of people you love who would appreciate an encouraging note. During your high-temptation times, write and mail a note instead of starting to eat.

- Make a list of things you love to do, need to do, or have been putting off. Write each one on a slip of paper. Fold them individually and put them in a pretty bowl or box. Next time you're tempted to overeat, pull one out and get busy.

- Sign up to do some volunteer work that would be fun and rewarding to you. Schedule it during your high-temptation times, if possible.

- Purchase a Bible study guide at a bookstore and begin a personal Bible study on a topic that interests you.

- Take a long walk, or do some other kind of exercise.
- Pray!

—CDC

Prayer

Father, I thank you for giving me the courage and the insight to change. Help me to weed the garden of my heart, to get rid of the habits and patterns that are holding me back. Lead me to alternative activities in times of temptation. Thank you, Lord, that there is always a "way of escape" from these times. Help me, Father, to find it and take it. In Jesus' name, Amen.

Scripture

But remember this—the wrong desires that come into your life aren't anything new and different. Many others have faced exactly the same problems before you. And no temptation is irresistible. You can trust God to keep the temptation from becoming so strong that you can't stand up against it, for he has promised this and will do what he says. He will show you how to escape temptation's power so that you can bear up patiently against it. (1 Corinthians 10:13 TLB)

Food for Thought

Changing our eating behaviors is very difficult, but change is easier when we learn to substitute a positive activity for a negative one.

ASSIGNMENTS

1. Make a chart of the times of day or occasions during which you are tempted to overeat. Next to each one, write out one or more alternative activities that you could do at these times instead of eating.

2. Stress can be one of the major triggers for overeating, and exercise is the ideal antidote to stress. Learn to recognize stress symptoms in yourself, and give yourself a dose of exercise. An exercise break might include stretching, stair climbing, or floor exercises, depending on where you are. You may wish to purchase an exercise DVD that you can pop in and exercise to for ten or fifteen minutes. These mini-workouts not only release physical tension but can also be great mood lifters!

3. Many of us have forgotten how to really have fun now that we are in the adult category. Planning some fun activity with an encouraging friend is an excellent alternative to eating. How long has it been since you've tried to roller-skate or bowl? An activity that also includes some form of exercise provides an added bonus.

day 6: attitudes and disciplines
order begets order

In my own life, order begets order. If I bring one small corner of my world into order (a dresser drawer, for instance, or a jewelry box), some magnetic dynamic is created that seems to draw other parts of my existence into that same field of organization.

Conversely, chaos begets chaos in my life. If I let some small thing slide (my correspondence or my laundry), other areas in my life will tumble after these until many, if not all, of my activities are affected.

My eating, like everything else, is affected by the order or disorder in my life. Healthy eating seems to follow order and organization in my life like an obedient puppy. Unhealthy overeating, on the other hand, trails after other forms of chaos in my life like an untidy and demanding child.

Something as simple as a written plan for the day can spare me needless forays into chaotic behavior. Annie Dillard has said that "a schedule defends from chaos and whim. It is a net for catching days . . . a peace and a haven set into the wreck of time."[2] When I spend a small amount of time each evening reviewing my commitments and selecting the priority items to do the next day, I'm way ahead when morning comes. If I spend thirty minutes to an hour each morning praising God, seeking his will, and giving him the hard stuff, my days (even the difficult ones) go more smoothly.

Planning is every bit as important in the area of eating. I used to have this saying scribbled on a piece of blue construction paper and tacked to my kitchen bulletin board: "Failing to plan is planning to fail." Heading out into a day full of unruly calories waiting to trip you up at every mealtime is foolhardy indeed! The time to make the important decisions about food is *before* it is heaped on a plate in front of you.

I know some people who write down every morsel of food they plan to eat the next day. Both Overeaters Anonymous and Overeaters Victorious (two weight-control support groups) recommend doing this. They further suggest sharing the daily food plan with a supportive friend or sponsor. These ideas have proved themselves invaluable to many people.

I tend to do a little better if I operate by *general* rather than specific guidelines. My general plan for eating might include such simple points as the following: (1) no sweets or snack foods, (2) no eating between meals, (3) moderate helpings at meals, and (4) no second helpings. Within these general limits, I can usually make good, healthy choices without feeling terribly hemmed in. Special occasions like a party or dinner at a restaurant need not throw me for a loop. I may decide to plan a healthy snack before a party to take the edge off my appetite. Or I may suggest a restaurant that prepares food compatible with my eating program.

One of the benefits of planning is the joy we experience as our eating behaviors begin to become more tame and orderly.

As this happens, we may be surprised to notice that other areas of our lives are becoming more orderly as well.

—CDC

Prayer

Father, I thank you that you are a God of order. You long for us to experience the joy of peaceful and orderly living. We submit our lives to you, asking you to bring order out of chaos. Teach us ways of serenity. Be our Guide as we learn to plan, and be our Source of power as we seek to follow the plans we have made. In Jesus' name we pray, Amen.

Scripture

Depend on the Lord in whatever you do,
and your plans will succeed. (Proverbs 16:3)

Food for Thought

Failing to plan is planning to fail.

ASSIGNMENTS

1. You may wish to include a calendar in the Planning section of your notebook with a separate page for each day. (Office supply stores sell these inserts for different-sized notebooks.) Using your calendar, spend time in the morning, the evening, or both prayerfully planning what you will do and what you will eat each day.

2. The fruit of the Spirit listed in Galatians 5:23 includes the fruit of "self-control," which can also be translated "self-discipline." God wishes to add order to our lives that we may operate in peace and harmony with him and others. Ask him to begin manifesting this quality in your life and surroundings as well as in your eating.

3. Stop and take an inventory of your progress in exercise. Has your daily workout become a regular part of your schedule? As disciplined exercise becomes second nature to you, it will encourage discipline in your eating as well.

4. Check your TV guide for exercise programs in your area. Mark on your calendar those programs that appeal to you, and purpose to keep those appointments. Keep researching programs or DVDs until you find one that works for you.

day 7: attitudes and disciplines
no excuse for excuses

My four-year-old friend William has a very active imagination. Last week he let it get away from him, and he told his carpool driver that he could read. When she asked for a demonstration, William realized immediately that he was in big trouble. He gazed thoughtfully out of the window for a moment before replying, "I'm sorry. I can't read and talk at the same time!"

Some of us imaginative types are just born with the gift of excuse-making. Take me, for instance. I have spent the past two months eating exactly what I want when I want it, which is too much too often. But the very imaginative excuse I have devised for the resulting weight gain is that I can't find time to exercise.

With an active toddler and a crowded schedule, that much is true. There is no time to exercise. But what exactly does that have to do with how much I've been eating? Watch carefully as the experienced excuse-maker answers that last question. The logic goes something like this: if you can't do *one*, why do *either*?

Yes, I really said that to myself. And yes, I even let myself believe it for a time. Maybe you're totally amazed that a sensible person could fall for such an illogical scam, and a self-inflicted one at that! Or maybe you recognize yourself as a fellow excuse-maker.

When we're finally serious, really serious, about changing our eating habits and attitudes, excuses have to go. What is cute in a four-year-old is the kiss of death to a reforming adult.

As I began to unmask my excuse, here was the truth I discovered: if I can't do both (exercise *and* eat right), then I can do one. I can concentrate my energy on learning to eat right. I can submit myself to God's training in making honest, healthy choices. I can commit myself to his plan for my daily menus. I can pray that I will eat food for the use, not the abuse, of my body.

And somehow I have the feeling that if I take care of one, God will take care of the other. If I am obedient in the area I can control, he will take control of the other. I know that all progress begins with that first small step. Here goes!

—LRB

Prayer
Father, you are a God of great mercy and quick compassion, and I confess to you that I am a person of greedy appetite and ready excuses. Forgive me for not stepping into the grace that you have in abundance for me. Put my feet back on the path of righteousness, one step at a time. Only you, Holy Spirit, can lead me and empower me to choose according to your will and your plan. Help me to desire only your best for me. In Jesus' name, Amen.

Scripture
You deserve honesty from the heart; yes, utter sincerity and truthfulness. Oh, give me this wisdom. (Psalm 51:6 TLB)

Food for Thought

When we're finally serious, really serious, about changing our eating habits and attitudes, excuses have to go.

ASSIGNMENTS

1. Ask God to show you any area that is preventing you from following your plan for healthy eating. Ask him to reveal to you any excuses to which you have been resorting. Write out your insights in the Journal section of your notebook. Pray that his Holy Spirit will empower you to confess and move on.

2. As you work out today, quote to yourself, "He gives me new strength. / He leads me on paths that are right / for the good of his name" (Ps. 23:3).

3. Share with your buddy (or a safe friend) the areas in which you have been making excuses. Ask that person to hold you accountable in these areas.

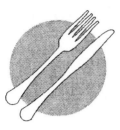

afterword
looking to the future

It's hard to believe you're here at the end of your six-week commitment. Congratulations are in order! Certainly by now you are noticing some real changes in your thought and behavior patterns where food and exercise are concerned. Hopefully your appearance is also reflecting those changes.

But this ending is really the beginning. All that you have learned and absorbed can be valuable only if you continue on the positive path you have charted for yourself. The principles you have taken time and care to acquire are lifetime investments.

Two of the most frequently played themes in Scripture are faithfulness and endurance. "We must not become tired of doing good," Paul cautioned the early Christians in Galatians 6:9. For it is to the faithful that the Lord promises a "crown of life" (Rev. 2:10).

Stephen W. Brown, who addressed the 1989 annual meeting of the Gospel Music Association in Nashville, pointed out that faithfulness can be measured not by what the world sees us doing, but by what we do when no one else is around. He gave a dramatic example of faithfulness by relating the story of the sculptor who designed the Statue of Liberty in New York Harbor.

Someone asked the sculptor why he was bothering to create the hair on top of the statue's head in such elaborate detail when no one would ever see it. (At that time, airplanes had not even been invented, and no one could have possibly foreseen the fact that people would indeed someday be flying over those intricate curls every day of the year!) The sculptor's answer to that question tells us a lot about the kind of person he was.

He answered simply, "God will know, and I will know." More than the approval of others, this man of integrity required the inner satisfaction of knowing that he was doing his best.

The Lord calls us to this kind of faithfulness as we continue our commitment to a lifetime of healthy eating. He desires the kind of quiet integrity that helps us persevere in doing what we know to be right. As David observed in Psalm 51, "Behold, thou desirest truth in the inward parts: and in the hidden part thou shalt make me to know wisdom" (v. 6 KJV).

But Jesus explained to his followers in John 13:17 that knowing what is right is only the first part of God's equation for a life of peace and purpose. "You know these things—now do them!" he said. "That is the path of blessing" (TLB).

For this reason, we not only congratulate you this day; we also challenge you to continue practicing the good habits and attitudes you have worked so hard to acquire.

- Continue surrendering to God's will for you one day at a time, seeking his wisdom and strength as you go.
- Continue making "the better choice" one day, one meal, one moment at a time.
- Continue to eat only when you are hungry and stop when you are comfortably full, not stuffed.

- Continue to share your personal journey with the Lord in your quiet time through prayer and journaling.
- Continue to study God's Word, relating his truth to your specific problems.
- Continue to gain strength from your supportive relationships.
- Continue regular exercise.

We firmly believe that God's plans for your future are more exciting and fulfilling than you can even begin to imagine. They are plans "to prosper you and not to harm you . . . to give you hope and a future" (Jer. 29:11 NIV). Our prayers go with you as you move into the excitement of this promise. We know that with his help and by his power, you are already in the process of overcoming every obstacle on the way.

Overcomers

If David killed Goliath with nothing but a stone,
If Daniel faced the lions' den with faith and faith alone,
If Moses and the Israelites just walked right through the sea,
Then God can overcome through you and me.

Chorus:
We're overcomers, by the power of the Son.
The fight's already won before we start.
We're overcomers, through what the Lord has done:
He put his overcoming love inside our hearts.

Now, Jesus beat the devil back with nothing but the Word,
And the walls of Jericho fell down when Joshua's shout was heard,
And we can tear down strongholds, too, if we have faith to see
That God can overcome through you and me.

Repeat chorus

Bridge:
He works his works through simple men and women
Who have the faith to take him at his Word,
And the power of the Spirit that raised Jesus from the dead
Lives in us to overcome this world!

Repeat chorus

—Claire Cloninger and Morris Chapman

appendix
personal inventory guide

1. Where am I now, and where would I like to be, in the area of
   - my weight?
   - my measurements?
   - my muscle tone?
   - my eating habits, behavior, etc.?
   - my exercise habits?
   - my appearance?
   - my general health?

2. How do my weight, appearance, eating habits, exercise, and general health affect:
   - my self-esteem?
   - my relationship with God?
   - my relationships with (list specific people or categories of relationships)?
   - my job, school, or other life work?

3. What do I hope to accomplish in the next forty days:
   - spiritually?
   - physically?
   - other?

notes

week one

1. Rebecca Manley Pippert, *Hope Has Its Reasons* (San Francisco: Harper & Row, 1989), 14.

week two

1. Jane Hirschmann and Carol H. Munter, *Overcoming Overeating* (New York: Ballantine, 1988), 9.
2. Geneen Roth, *Breaking Free from Compulsive Eating* (Bergefield, N.J.: New American Library, 1984), 177.

week three

1. Jeanie Miley, *Creative Silence* (Dallas, TX: Word, 1988).
2. Henry Nouwen, *The Way of the Heart* (New York: Ballantine, 1981), 8.

week five

1. Henry David Thoreau, *Thoreau on Man and Nature* (New York: Peter Pauper Press, 1960), 11.

week six

1. *Food for Thought*, Harper/Hazelden and Winston Press, 1980, Nov. 26.
2. Annie Dillard, *The Writing Life* (New York: Harper & Row, 1989), 32.